TOTAL HEALTH PROMOTION
Mental Health, Rational Fields and the Quest for Autonomy

David Seedhouse

Auckland University of Technology, New Zealand and Middlesex University, London, UK

JOHN WILEY & SONS LTD

Telephone (+44) 1243 779777

Email (for orders and customer service enquiries): cs-books@wiley.co.uk
Visit our Home Page on www.wileyeurope.com or www.wiley.com

Other Wiley Editorial Offices

John Wiley & Sons Inc., 111 River Street, Hoboken, NJ 07030, USA

Jossey-Bass, 989 Market Street, San Francisco, CA 94103-1741, USA

Wiley-VCH Verlag GmbH, Boschstr. 12, D-69469 Weinheim, Germany

John Wiley & Sons Australia Ltd, 33 Park Road, Milton, Queensland 4064, Australia

John Wiley & Sons (Asia) Pte Ltd, 2 Clementi Loop #02-01, Jin Xing Distripark, Singapore 129809

John Wiley & Sons Canada Ltd, 22 Worcester Road, Etobicoke, Ontario, Canada M9W 1L1

British Library Cataloguing in Publication Data

A catalogue record for this book is available from the British Library

ISBN 0 471 49013 X

Typeset in 10/12 Palatino from the author's disks by Dobbie Typesetting Limited, Tavistock, Devon
Printed and bound in Great Britain by Antony Rowe Ltd, Chippenham, Wiltshire
This book is printed on acid-free paper responsibly manufactured from sustainable forestry in which at least two trees are planted for each one used for paper production.

Contents

Preface

> All progress is initiated by challenging current conceptions, and executed by supplanting existing institutions. Consequently, the first condition of progress is the removal of all censorships.
>
> (George Bernard Shaw, Preface to *Mrs. Warren's Profession*, 1893*)

There are different kinds of censorship. There are deliberate prohibitions, there are unspoken taboos, and then there are all those ways in which we unthinkingly censor ourselves. This book is about the latter. In particular, it is about how we censor our ethical imagination as we complacently accept comfortable classifications of the world.

We have to classify reality. Without classification we merely prowl the earth. The only way we can move beyond instinct is to distinguish one bit of meaning from another. So we separate highbrow hobbies from popular culture, childhood from adulthood, intelligence from stupidity, sanity from madness – and make a million other conceptual divisions, mapping the world as we want to see it. But as soon as we come to believe our classifications are real like rock is real we are trapped. We could see the world as a perpetual adventure, but instead we bury ourselves under a heap of conventions, unwilling and unable to find the strength to shake them off.

Evidence of self-inflicted censorship is all around us. Opinion polls repeatedly show that the majority of us make concrete divisions between criminals and regular people, terrorists and non-terrorists, social status and social disgrace, leisure and work, friends and strangers. We seem compelled to plaster the world with labels: organic and non-organic food, natural and unnatural environments, national airspace and international airspace – we even stuck flags on the moon. Most of us think our classifications *really* exist – we believe criminals would be criminals even if there were no lawmakers, that terrorists are terrorists as a matter of fact, and that work and leisure are absolutely different activities – just as impermeable as they felt when most of us had to clock on and off for the day. But these things are only as real as we want them to be. We are so used to talking about mental illness, twists of fate, and the dignity of nations (no matter how vicious they are to each other) that we assume such things are as real as grass and rain and ice. But they are not. We make the decision to arrange the evidence under these headings. We design the labels, and we tie them to the world.

Conventional health promotion makes hundreds of artificial distinctions. Health promotion textbooks differentiate between responsible and irresponsible behaviour, safe and unsafe practices, more and less risky actions, disease and health, subjective and objective well-being, mental health and physical health – and always the assumption is

---

*Acknowledgement to the Society of Authors' on behalf of the George Bernard Shaw Estate.

that these different categories exist independently of the choice to classify them. But it is just not true. In every case pieces of evidence – of behaviour, of state of mind, of physical process – are shaped according to our interpretations of them.

All human conventions have the potential both to enable and to restrict us. I am writing this Preface on Boxing Day, 2001. For the last few weeks, people all over the world have been roped into Christmas, like it or not. They have had to buy presents, to go to parties, to be jolly to each other, to wear Santa hats and red reindeer antlers, to visit relatives they have no interest in, and to eat and drink more than they usually do. Some people love this sort of thing. Some of us hate it. But whatever we feel, it is very hard to escape it altogether.

Most of the ways we organise the world have the same effect. Some people love them, some people hate them, most of us tolerate them, and very few of us seem able to change even the tiniest bit of them. When we detest a particular part of the social world we know intuitively what is wrong – we have been channelled into ways of behaving against our will, but we can't properly explain how, and so we can't work out how to break free.

And yet there are escape routes open to all of us, so long as we are prepared to see convention for what it is. Instead of thinking and behaving according to established rules and patterns, we can analyse their structure. And when we do it is easy to see that our conventions are rational fields. Like all other manifestations of life, our social habits are purposive systems made up of goals, strategies and means (a plant stretching for light is a rational field, a person seeking a new job creates a rational field, a health promotion plan is a rational field). Seen like this, we can immediately ask searching questions about our rational fields. Why this goal? Does this goal fit with that one? Why not this goal instead? Is this the best strategy? What about its unwanted effects? What are the alternatives? Is this the best we can achieve with these means? Is the present system the most ethical option? Might different rational fields create greater health?

Once you realise that rational fields are everywhere not only can you begin to choose between them, but you can deliberately form as many new ones as your creativity allows. All you need to do is define goals and have the means and open-mindedness to find the most effective strategies to reach them – it is quite immaterial whether or not these goals and methods are listed in the *Manual of Official Classifications*.

Total Health Promotion is an argument for the removal of self-censorship, but it does not condemn all conventions. Most of them stem from a hard-to-undo mix of classifications and reality *per se*, and many are productive and sensible. However, it does ask that we exercise the power to reflect creatively on all our social compulsions, and it explains why and how we should act to change those that are not as health promoting as they could be.

Total Health Promotion takes two widely used, conventional classifications – psychiatry and mental health – and demonstrates that they are speculations at best. These examples are used to show that if we can find the courage to cast thoughtless health promotion distinctions aside, we are free to establish total health promotion – an intellectually liberated yet practically focused devotion to human autonomy.

David Seedhouse
Auckland
Christmas, 2001

Acknowledgements

I have only myself to blame for this work. As I write, no one has commented on it. In fact no one else has even seen it yet, so I can truly say that all its philosophical mistakes and stylistic flaws are my own.

Nevertheless, I hope that its obvious enthusiasm – though undoubtedly naïve and error-full – will prove to be a catalyst for a more open, creative and philosophically substantial form of health promotion. *Total Health Promotion* is so confident about itself that it must surely provoke a reaction, even from the most stick-in-the-mud health promoter.

Though they had nothing at all to do with its words and pictures, I would like to thank my wife and daughters, and my colleagues at Auckland University of Technology, Middlesex University and John Wiley & Sons Ltd, for their friendship and support during the writing of this book.

Introduction

By any stretch of the imagination, this is not a traditional health promotion book. There is no mention of health promotion models and standards, it has nothing to say about epidemiology or lifestyle management, and there is not even a sniff of a health promotion target to be found within its pages. If you are looking for a conventional exposition of the merits of health promotion, this is not the book for you. However, if you want to understand how health promotion might move beyond its fixation with disease and illness, and at last live up to its aspiration to provide meaningful health for all, then read on.

The trouble with conventional health promotion is that it is conventional. Conventional health promotion – the sort of health promotion that tells people to stop smoking cigarettes and drinking alcohol and cajoles us to get our kids immunised – uses traditional assumptions and traditional techniques. Because these assumptions and techniques are so well established amongst conventional health promoters, conventional health promotion finds it virtually impossible to conceive that they might be questionable.

The conventional health promotion industry – a vast, informal consortium of government administrators, public health officials, medical professionals, academics, researchers, practitioners and consumer movements – continues to expand. As it does so, it develops more and more specialist branches: public health, public safety, disease surveillance, family health, health in developing countries, heart health, child health, community development, well-being promotion, mental health promotion – the list goes on. Each new specialism strengthens conventional health promotion simply by adding to its chain-mail of conventions.

As a trained and instinctive philosopher, conventional health promotion has always filled me with disquiet. *My* assumption is that institutions unable to criticise themselves – and unable to see the point of criticisms made from outside their walls – are certainly less useful to us all than they might be, and are probably dangerous to at least some of us. I have explained this in detail in a previous work, *Health Promotion: Philosophy, Prejudice and Practice* (which may usefully be read alongside the present book), and had thought this was all I had to say on the subject.

The present book was originally meant to be entirely about mental health promotion. I imagined it would do a similar job to *Health Promotion: Philosophy, Prejudice and Practice*, this time with sole reference to the mental realm. I had in mind a book which would disentangle the ubiquitous muddles over the nature of mental illness and mental health, and assess the merits of various approaches to mental health promotion – psychiatry, psychology, mental morbidity prevention, well-being promotion, and alternatives to psychiatry – before offering a constructive way forward using the foundations theory of health, my own health promotion preference. But no sooner had I begun than I realised that this plan would have to be aborted. It dawned on me that not only are mental health and mental illness artificial categories – categories manufactured by human beings – but the distinction between the physical and mental realm is artificial too. Given this, I could not possibly write a book exclusively about mental health promotion.

So I wrote a different book. *Total Health Promotion* does discuss different understandings of 'the mental' (**Part One** may be read as a rough and ready review of contemporary beliefs about mental health and illness). But it does not do so to establish a case for best practice in mental health promotion. Rather it discusses mental health and illness in order to show how strange it is to divide the mental from the physical – despite the fact that most of us make the separation all the time.

The belief that the mental and the physical are entirely and forever apart is perpetuated almost everywhere in Western culture – in schools, in leisure activities, by Christianity, by the health professions, by the news media: by the very way we organise our social systems into compartments for 'mental stuff' (mental hospitals, psychiatry, counselling, intellectual intelligence, emotional intelligence) and 'physical stuff' (general hospitals, organic medicine, sport, physical health promotion, work 'with the hands' and so on).

We seem to think and feel emotion in our heads, and move and touch with our bodies, and so it seems only natural that we should have disciplines devoted to the health of our mental lives, and other quite separate disciplines devoted to the health of our physical organs, tissues and cells. But even though we routinely divide the world up like this, the mental/physical split is no more necessary than the idea that 'schools are where kids get educated' and 'outside school is where kids do non-educational things', or the idea that there are white people and there are black people and they are not the same. We make such classifications because they make sense to some of us – they offer some sort of explanation of our human experience, they appeal to some of our instincts, and some of us find the values they represent reassuring. We make them. They don't make themselves.

Total Health Promotion argues that once we countenance the possibility that we do not have to be bound by strict separations of the mental and the physical – and therefore no longer need to be glued into rigid specialisms like psychiatry, mental health promotion and strictly organic medicine – we are free to be infinitely creative in our health promotion activities. We do not, for instance, have to restrict ourselves (in a box labelled mental health promotion) to techniques designed to improve the 'maturity' or 'sense of self' of an individual with a mental disorder. Indeed, once liberated from fixed categories, we can see that it is better not to think of 'individuals with mental disorders' at all – because this classification inexorably binds us to a focus on the individual, or even to a focus on an individual's thought processes or brain function. It is far more liberating to concentrate on 'life difficulties', since the idea of life difficulties enables us to consider *either* the individual *or* the life circumstances surrounding the individual, or both.

Total health promoters should always endeavour to see the total picture – however conflicting it is and however difficult it may be to do so.

THE ARGUMENT

Total Health Promotion is an ambitious book, but it tries not to overreach itself. It offers a blueprint for a reflective, uninhibited form of health promotion, in the following simple steps.

CHAPTER ONE

The opening chapter argues that our urge to classify things and processes into distinct categories is an inescapable reaction to a world that is otherwise far too complicated for us to comprehend. We tend to think our classifications are discoveries – that we have found the world to be as we think it is. But we are mostly mistaken.

By means of a well-known mid-twentieth-century murder case – made notorious for a second time by the 1994 film *Heavenly Creatures* – Chapter One suggests that no matter how obviously right it looks to some of us, the statement 'this person is mentally ill' depends as much on beyond-the-evidence assumptions as the statements 'this person is possessed', 'this person is evil', and 'this person is criminal'.

CHAPTER TWO

Since Chapter One's conclusion is controversial – and will no doubt be rejected out of hand by most psychiatrists – Chapter Two shows that psychiatry would not exist without beyond-the-evidence assumptions, and explains that alternative classifications of mental problems are therefore equally as plausible as psychiatry's.

CHAPTER THREE

Chapter Three describes different definitions of mental health. It points out that just like classifications of mental illness, all understandings of mental health sit permanently beyond-the-evidence. Consequently, definitions of mental health are of little use for total health promotion, since each is artificially disconnected from the physical and social world.

CHAPTER FOUR

Chapter Four gives detailed reasons why we should not automatically separate the mental from the physical, and explains why it makes more sense to think of the world as fundamentally interconnected. In so doing the chapter begins to consolidate the groundwork for total health promotion.

CHAPTER FIVE

This chapter explains what rational fields are. It describes the difference between a natural rational field and a manufactured one, and it shows how a mix of evidence and non-evidence can be combined to create manufactured rational fields. Chapter Five also explains how to assess the stability of manufactured rational fields, using the examples of psychiatry and mental health promotion. In the process, it demonstrates that psychiatry and mental health promotion are both disintegrating rational fields, artificially held together by human instincts, values and classifications.

CHAPTER SIX

The final chapter explains three important steps. It shows how to analyse rational fields by asking ten clarifying questions (**STEP 1**). It explains how to compare and contrast rational fields in context (**STEP 2**). And it demonstrates how total health promoters can combine the foundations theory of health with rational field thinking, in order to devise the most thoughtful and practical health-promoting schemes (**STEP 3**).

As it works through these steps and explores different health promotion challenges, Chapter Six shows how health promotion could be released from its artificial conventions to become self-critical, ethically mature and focused on autonomy creation.

TOTAL HEALTH PROMOTION

I am under no illusions as I offer this book. Having been a health promoter myself for a while, I understand health promotion culture and am well aware of the pressure on working health promoters to conform to conventional expectations. I also realise that the book does not even look like a health promotion text, at least not in **Part One**. I imagine *Total Health Promotion* will be met with either incomprehension or miscomprehension by the bulk of its conventional health promotion audience (assuming there is an audience at all). However, even knowing this, I put the book forward in the belief that it is an important contribution to health promotion's future. I confess that the book is patchy, and I admit that the idea of using rational fields to promote health is underdeveloped and untried. Nonetheless, I think there is tremendous potential to refine this ground-breaking approach to health promotion.

If total health promotion were to become widely adopted the social advantage could be enormous. At present, most health promotion is conservative, unreflective and seeks to change people's behaviours by training us, indoctrinating us or passing laws to make us behave – and it usually does so without seeking individual or public consent. Conventional health promotion cannot see anything wrong with this approach, but total health promotion thinks quite differently. Where the conventional health promoter proceeds as a matter of course, the total health promoter reflects and analyses in ethical and practical detail, taking as little as possible for granted. Unlike conventional health promotion, total health promotion has wholly explicit purposes, and it uses a template that can be applied to assess any and all health promotion interventions. Crucially, this template demands absolute honesty about the instincts, values and classifications that must lie behind any health promotion plan.

PART ONE

Filing Reality

CHAPTER ONE

Beyond-the-Evidence

SUMMARY

This chapter:

- Discusses our urge to make sense of the world by classifying it in separate compartments
- Takes a notorious murder and attempts to understand why it happened
- Defines various types of evidence and non-evidence
- Explains that to make sense of the murder evidence alone is not enough – we must go beyond-the-evidence
- Argues that we resort to beyond-the-evidence assumptions and decisions more frequently than we commonly acknowledge
- Concludes that the statement 'this person is mentally ill' relies on beyond-the-evidence assumptions just as much as the statements 'this person is possessed', 'this person is evil', and 'this person is criminal'

HEAVENLY CREATURES: POSSESSED, EVIL, CRIMINAL OR ILL?

What does it take to make you kill your mother?

> Pauline had slipped the piece of brick into the foot of an old stocking, thus making an effective sling-shot. Juliet was 60 yards in front, and still out of sight down the track, when Honora Parker caught sight of a pink pebble, and Pauline remarked how pretty it was. Honora bent down to pick it up. Behind her, Pauline pulled the sling-shot from her pocket, braced her legs, and swung. The brick crashed on her mother's head, and she collapsed. And that was the moment when Pauline wished it hadn't happened. But some force possessed her, drove her on, some inner voice which commanded: It is too late to stop! She struck again, and again, and now Juliet, panting from a sprint along the track, was kneeling beside her, and swinging the sling-shot. Blood was spurting from twenty-four wounds in Honora Parker's face and head. Sobbing hysterically, the girls looked at each other and at their victim. The blood was only trickling now. They had beaten Honora Mary Parker to death.[1]

Pauline was 16 and Juliet 15 when they murdered Honora Parker. Even in our numbingly violent world, when teenage girls kill a parent it is safe to say something's gone wrong. But what was it? What caused the girls to behave like this?

THE EVIDENCE

There's no doubt about the evidence. According to Mr Brown, the Crown prosecutor:

> 'About 3.30 p.m. on the afternoon of June 22 (1954), two girls came running into the tearooms (in Victoria Park, Christchurch, New Zealand) agitated, breathless, and gasping, "Please help us. Mummy has been hurt – covered with blood." A few minutes later, the body of Mrs Parker was found, her head terribly battered. The situation of her body and the gross injuries to her head were so unusual that the police were called, and it was quickly apparent that she had been killed by being brutally battered about the head with a brick... That evening, Pauline Parker was arrested, and the next day her close friend Juliet Hulme was arrested. The evidence will make it terribly clear that these two young accused conspired together to kill the mother of one of them, and horribly carried their plan into effect.'[2]

Rupert Furneaux continues the story in *Famous Criminal Cases*, again in the words of Mr Brown:

> 'The evidence will be that the two accused came to the conclusion, after much thought, that the mother of the accused Parker was an obstacle in their path, that she thwarted their desires and that she should be done away with...
>
> 'Pauline Parker and Juliet Hulme met at school and became friendly and this friendship developed into an intense devotion. Their main object in life was to be together, sharing each other's thoughts, secrets and plans, and if any person dared to part them, then that person should be forcibly removed. Mrs. Parker became perturbed at the unhealthy relationship and tried to break it up. This was resented by the accused and the resentment gradually grew into hate and eventually resulted in this ghastly crime.
>
> 'Early in 1954 Dr. Hulme, who had resigned his position as Rector of Canterbury University College, decided to return to England and to take his daughter Juliet to South Africa. It was discovered that the two girls were planning to go to America to have their novels published and that they had tried to acquire funds to pay their fares. Both girls were determined not to be parted, and Pauline Parker wanted to go to South Africa and Juliet Hulme wanted her to go with her. Both girls knew that Mrs. Parker would be the one to object most strenuously to their going away together. They decided the best way to end Mrs. Parker's objection was to kill her in such a manner that it would appear to have been an accident.
>
> 'Early in June when the date of Dr. Hulme's departure had been fixed for 3rd July, the girls coldly and calculatingly formed a plan to kill Mrs. Parker. They pretended to be resigned to being parted and they persuaded her to take them for a farewell outing. They planned to entice her to a secluded spot and strike her on the head. They would then rush for help, announcing that she had died as a result of a fall.
>
> 'On the day of the outing Juliet Hulme took with her part of a brick from her home. After the accident they both told the same story.'[3]

Furneaux expands:

> Mr. Brown next described the finding of Pauline Parker's diary. 'In it,' he said, 'she reveals that she and Juliet Hulme have engaged in shoplifting, toyed with blackmail and talked about and played with matters of sex. There is clear evidence that as long ago as February

> she was anxious that her mother should die and that during the few weeks before 22nd June she was planning to kill her mother in the way she was killed.'
>
> Extracts of the diary were read in court.
>
> 13th February: Why could not mother die? Dozens of people, thousands of people are dying every day. So why not mother, and father too?
> 28th April: Anger against mother boiled up inside me. It is she who is one of the main obstacles in my path. Suddenly a means of ridding myself of the obstacle occurred to me.
> 29th April: I did not tell Deborah (her pet name for Juliet) of my plans for removing mother... the last fate I wish to meet is one in a Borstal. ...I am trying to think of some way. I want it to appear either a natural or an accidental death.
> 19th June: We practically finished our books (the novels the girls were writing together) today and our main 'ike' for the day was to moider mother. The notion is not a new one, but this time it is a definite plan which we intend to carry out. We have worked it out carefully and are both thrilled with the idea. Naturally we feel a trifle nervous, but the pleasure of anticipation is great.
> 20th June: We discussed our plans for moidering mother and made them a little clearer. Peculiarly enough I have no qualms of conscience (or is it peculiar we are so mad?).
> 21st June: We decided to use a brick in a stocking rather than a sandbag. We discussed the moider fully. I feel keyed up as if I was planning a surprise party. So next time I write in the diary mother will be dead. How odd, yet how pleasing.
> 22nd June: I am writing a little of this up in the morning before the death. I felt very excited and the night before Christmassy last night. I did not have pleasant dreams though.[3]

Juliet's mother provided a little more insight into the girls' thinking:

> Mrs. Hulme described how the two girls wrote to each other in the characters of the stories that they were writing together. Juliet was first Charles II, Emperor of Borovnia. Then she became Deborah, the Emperor's mistress by whom she had a son, Dialbo [sic]. Pauline Parker started as Lancelot Trelawney, a soldier of fortune, and he succeeds in wedding the Empress of Bolumnia and becomes Emperor, and they have a daughter, Mariole. Pauline assumed these characters in turn and wrote to Juliet as such. The earlier part of the correspondence, she said, is extravagant and grandiose but it later becomes suicide and sudden death [sic]. Later violence and bloodshed figure to a disproportionate degree.[3]

MOVING BEYOND THE EVIDENCE

The story so far is unequivocal: the girls killed Honora Parker with a brick, Pauline Parker kept a diary in which she explained the murder plan, the plan went wrong, the girls were arrested and charged with murder. This much just is evidence – historical events it makes no sense to doubt. However, as soon as we try to make sense of the events, certainty dissolves into speculation. There is the unadorned evidence, there are interpretations of the evidence and – as the philosopher David Hume famously noted – these are of quite different epistemological standing:

> Take any action allow'd to be vicious: Wilful murder, for instance. Examine it in all lights, and see if you can find that matter of fact, or real existence, which you call *vice*. You can never find it, 'till you turn your reflexion into your own breast, and find a sentiment of disapprobation, which arises in you toward this action.[4]

Hume was referring to moral judgements only. However, his insight applies in general to other human interpretations, particularly though not exclusively to those made in the social realm. More often than not, the evidence does not speak for itself. What matters is what we make of it.

PSYCHIATRY BEYOND-THE-EVIDENCE

In the trial of Pauline and Juliet, different sets of psychiatrists examined exactly the same evidence and came to entirely opposed conclusions, not only about the girls' morality but also about their clinical, social and legal status:

> ...both defence counsel, Mr. Gresson for Hulme and Dr. Haslam for Parker, addressed the court. Mr. Gresson said that the fact that Parker and Hulme assaulted [Mrs. Parker] and killed her is, unfortunately, clear beyond dispute. ...He said that he would call witnesses who would say that Parker and Hulme were insane when they committed their attack on [Mrs. Parker], and were still suffering from a mental illness known as paranoia of the exalted type associated with *folie à deux*, a phrase meaning communicated insanity. He concluded: 'The Crown has seen fit to refer to the accused as ordinary, dirty-minded little girls. Our evidence will show that they are nothing of the kind. The Crown's description is unfortunate and medically incorrect. They are mentally sick girls, more to be pitied than blamed.'[3]
>
> Dr. Reginald Medlicott was also called by the defence. He told the court that when he...interviewed the girls in prison they constantly abused him. 'Parker told me I was an irritating fool and displeasing to look at. Hulme pulled me over the coals for not talking sufficiently clearly. After I had physically examined Parker she shouted out, "I hope you break your flaming neck".'
>
> 'There was,' he said, 'a gross reversal of moral sense. They admired those things which are evil and condemned those things the community considers good. They had weird ideas and their own paradise, god and religion.'
>
> He read to the court a poem, 'The Ones That I Worship,' composed by the girls:
>
> There are living amongst us two dutiful daughters
> Of a man who possesses two beautiful daughters
> The most glorious beings in creation
> They'd be the pride and joy of any nation.
> You cannot know nor try to guess
> The sweet soothingness of their caress.
> The outstanding genius of this pair
> Is understood by few, they are so rare.
> Compared with these two every man is a fool,
> The world is most honoured that they should deign to rule
> And above us these goddesses reign on high.
> I worship the power of these lovely two
> With that adoring love known to so few.
> 'Tis indeed a miracle one must feel,
> That two such heavenly creatures are real.
> Both sets of eyes, though different far, hold many mysteries strange
> Impassively they watch the race of man decay and change.
> Hatred burning bright in the brown eyes with enemies for fuel.
> Icy scorn glitters in the grey eyes, contemptuous and cruel.
> Why are men such fools they will not realise
> The wisdom that is hidden behind those strange eyes?
> And these wonderful people are you and I.
>
> 'The whole thing' said Dr. Medlicott 'rises to a fantastic crescendo. In my opinion they were insane when they attacked [Mrs. Parker].'[3]

Dr Kenneth Stallworthy – for the prosecution – disagreed:

> 'I consider them sane medically because I did not consider either certifiable, and I consider them sane in a legal sense. They knew the nature and quality of their act. I am of the

> opinion that they both knew at the time that their action was wrong in law, and that they were breaking the law. In the diaries there was evidence of motive, planning and premeditation.'[3]

Two other doctors called by the prosecution, Dr Saville and Dr Hunter, also believed the girls were sane.

This apparently bizarre state of affairs – psychiatrists at loggerheads over the single thing about which they are supposed to be expert – is a phenomenon that persists as much now as ever.[5] Some critics claim that such fundamental conflict shows that psychiatry is worthless.[6] But things are a little more complicated than this – if psychiatry is worthless because it depends on untestable judgements about the evidence then so is the great majority of human intellectual endeavour.

The doctors for the defence and prosecution found it impossible to agree not because the whole of psychiatry is meaningless (it is obviously meaningful to most psychiatrists and many patients), but because most human knowledge depends on beyond-the-evidence assumptions.[7] This is true of psychiatry (all judgements about mental illness are made according to an unprovable diagnostic system invented by human beings). It is true of the law (judges must interpret the meaning of cases and statutes, and often do so in contradictory ways).[8] And it is also true of much scientific activity:

> The process of scientific inquiry seldom delivers definitive answers about the nature of complicated psychological phenomena. Empirical findings are usually piecemeal fragments of a wider picture, and researchers must make choices about how to interpret the sometimes contradictory findings, both in relation to each other and with respect to existing explanatory frameworks. Given the complexity and indeterminacy of this process, there is always room for researchers' moral and political interests to influence conclusions they draw from the empirical evidence...[9]

Neither in law nor in psychiatry or psychology is it possible to resolve disputes about different interpretations of the evidence entirely by appeal to the evidence itself. As in the Heavenly Creatures' trial, once the unadorned evidence is clear it has no further role – everything of importance after that is beyond-the-evidence. And beyond-the-evidence interpretations can only be resolved by beyond-the-evidence means, which are many and diverse and include logic, reason, politics, expedience, majority decision, coercion, peer pressure and other human devices.

Figure 1 shows a simplified version of the relationship between the unadorned evidence and beyond-the-evidence interpretations in the Heavenly Creatures case. Inside the circle there is evidence – physical data, diaries, eyewitness statements, photographs of Honora Parker's injuries etc. – all of it raw material that would continue to exist if the human race became extinct at this very moment. Many things can be resolved entirely within the circle: were the physical signs consistent with attack by a brick? Was the blood on the sock Honora Parker's? What are the penalties for murder? What do the diaries say? However, sooner or later the evidence alone is not enough. To understand *why* the girls murdered Honora we have no choice but to stand outside the circle of evidence.

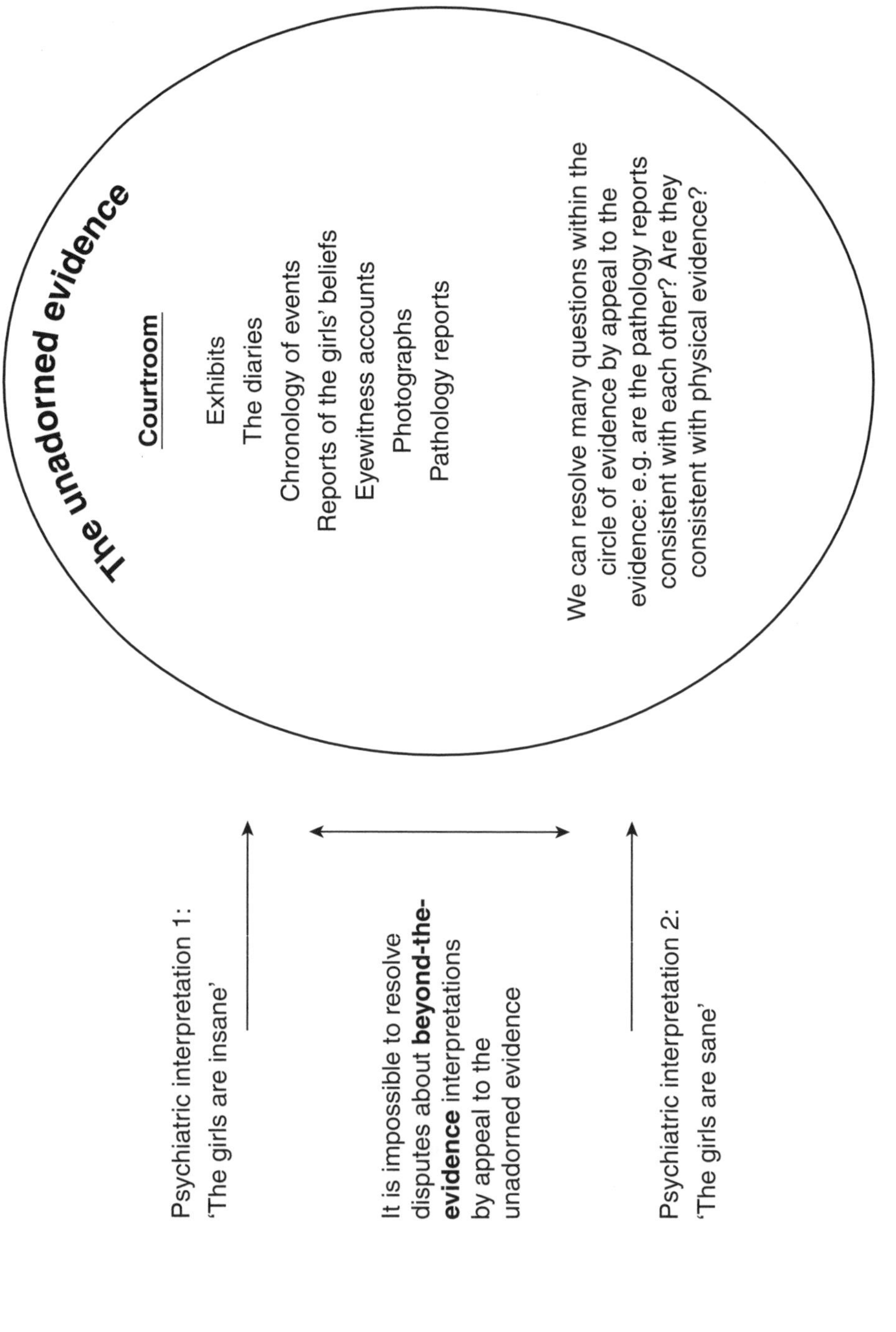
The unadorned evidence
Courtroom
Exhibits
The diaries
Chronology of events
Reports of the girls' beliefs
Eyewitness accounts
Photographs
Pathology reports
We can resolve many questions within the circle of evidence by appeal to the evidence: e.g. are the pathology reports consistent with each other? Are they consistent with physical evidence?
Psychiatric interpretation 1:
'The girls are insane'
It is impossible to resolve disputes about beyond-the-evidence interpretations by appeal to the unadorned evidence
Psychiatric interpretation 2:
'The girls are sane'

Figure 1 A simple picture of within and beyond-the-evidence interpretations in the Heavenly Creatures case

THE PLACE OF EVIDENCE AND NON-EVIDENCE IN THE WAY WE MAKE SENSE OF THE WORLD

Types of evidence and non-evidence can be distinguished as follows:

WITHIN-THE-EVIDENCE

Type 1: It just is
Generally speaking, there are certain events and processes that **just are**. In the Heavenly Creatures case: the woman once known as Honora Parker is dead, a murder trial took place in Christchurch in 1954, brick can break bone if it is wielded forcibly enough.

Type 2: Testable speculations
There are speculations that can be tested by reference to the **just is** evidence – for example, 'this brick has Honora Parker's blood on it', 'these injuries were not caused by an accidental fall', 'the girls wrote emotionally intense letters to each other' – each of which can be confirmed or denied by means of the evidence. Theory is usually required to confirm this sort of speculation (in the Heavenly Creatures case theories about blood typing, causes of injury, and psychology are needed in addition to the unadorned evidence) but ultimately it is the evidence that establishes or refutes the speculation.

BEYOND-THE-EVIDENCE

When the evidence will not yield the explanations we require, we must move beyond-the-evidence. As we do so we resort to:

Type 3: Speculations that cannot currently be tested
Our speculations may be untestable:

(a) Because we do not yet have adequate techniques to do the tests (for example, we might speculate that only Pauline swung the brick, but we have no means to confirm this independently, and must therefore accept the girls' word that they both hit Mrs Parker).
(b) Because reality is too complex for us to determine whether our speculations are correct (for example, we might believe that a brain abnormality was the root cause of the murder, but never be able to prove it because the interplay between brains and the social world defies human comprehension).

Type 4: Speculations that cannot in principle be tested
'Satanic possession caused the girls to kill their mother' and 'it was pre-destined that the girls would kill their mother' are both examples of this type, since both beliefs are essentially matters of faith.

Type 5: Human classifications – ways of filing reality
Type 5 is an important, pervasive and yet undernoticed feature of human life. Not

only do we continually make both instinctive and intentional beyond-the-evidence decisions to classify evidence into categories, but we must do so if we are to make any sense of things at all.

We have to classify the world in order to think about it and act in it. For instance, unless we demarcate desirable behaviour from antisocial behaviour, normal thinking from abnormal thinking, and illness from non-illness – and make countless other daily distinctions – we are powerless to negotiate our social environment.

Many of our classifications stem directly from the evidence. For example, it **just is** the case that certain types of animal cannot reproduce with other types of animal. We have chosen to label these reproductive groups 'species', a decision which assists us in other speculations about biology and evolution.[10] It also **just is** the case that heavy bodies are attracted to the earth. We assume there must be an invisible force at work, which we call gravity – a classification that seems to help us understand some of the workings of the universe.[11] And of course we have created taxonomies of disease (infection by microorganism, for example) that directly reflect the evidence as it **just is**.

The trouble is that we tend to believe that classifications (like sanity and insanity) that stem from beyond-the-evidence are just as certain as those (like sentient and non-sentient) that come from within it – they can seem to us to be just as factual as the laws of biology and physics. In Western societies, for example, 'family' (meaning Mum, Dad, the children and a few close relatives) is commonly thought of as a unit of reality – something that just exists. And yet it is very obviously we who name different collections of individuals. We take the unadorned evidence of relationship (be it blood group, genetics, physical resemblance or merely geographical proximity) and label it 'family'. But this label does not exist outside human convention. As everyone knows, 'family' has different meanings in different cultures – for example, Maori consider family to be *whanau* or *Iwi* (far broader notions than the typical Western one).

'Intelligence' is conventionally defined as a capacity to understand verbal nuance, visual pattern and mathematical relationship. This classification has become so enshrined in Western culture that whole careers can depend on how well one does in intelligence tests. However, there is no reason other than convention why artistic skill, poetic ability, the ability to empathise, or musical talent should not be considered the essence of intelligence. Educational philosophers, for example, define a variety of *intelligences* – linguistic, logical, musical, spatial, bodily, inter- and intrapersonal, amongst others – challenging the assumption that intelligence is something that can be measured by a conventional IQ test.[12]

Intelligence is not a unit of reality, intelligence is what we say it is. And the same is true of many other segments of the world we have chosen to categorise. It is even true of 'addiction':

> Since the eighteenth century, western man has organised particular behaviours into a specific, unitary phenomenon – namely, 'addiction' – as if this combination of behaviours is a distinct and real entity. The reasons why this combination of behaviours is created is not different from the reasons why the behavioural entity

> 'possessed by the devil' was created as the by-product of a past, religious, world view.... 'Addiction' is easily recognised by the culturally initiated, in the same way as in voodoo the impact of particular Spirits is recognised out of behavioural elements that a non-initiated person would not even see, or would understand in a completely different way.[13]

Addiction exists as a category because we have taken some features of the world, seen them as significant, and lumped them together into a parcel that makes sense for us, at our time and in our culture. Of course some people develop habits and crave for one thing or another. But – like all the hundreds of other supposed mental illnesses – addiction exists as a category mainly because we want it to – it is an explanation that in some way fits with the evidence, and in some way suits us.

We are surrounded by an endless tangle of undefined processes, events and things – and we are driven to make sense of them: we are irresistibly programmed to be the world's librarians. We file reality – as diseases, as illnesses, as measurements, as work, as leisure, as dates, as chunks of time, as charity, as right and wrong: we take the evidence, we decide its significance, we make it meaningful.

Type 6: How we value the evidence

Whether we realise it or not, we continually interpret the evidence in accord with our moral preferences. And the way we value the evidence in turn affects and is affected by our speculations and classifications. For example, we may believe that human beings are entirely responsible for our actions (a **Type 4** speculation that cannot in principle be tested by reference to the evidence), that we should therefore be held accountable for these actions (a **Type 5** judgement that there is accountability and non-accountability and a **Type 6** judgement that it is good to hold people to account), and that we should be punished – as criminals – for unacceptable actions (a **Type 5** classification between criminals and non-criminals and a **Type 6** judgement that criminals ought to be punished). Or we may hold that sometimes people become mentally ill (a **Type 5** judgement) and – when we do become ill – that we should not be held responsible for our actions (judgements of **Type 5** and **6**).

Type 7: Techniques of analysis

When we use reason and logic to consider the evidence we are not using the evidence itself – rather we are using beyond-the-evidence techniques to assess it. And the same applies to political techniques, coercion and all our other manipulations of each other.

Type 8: Defining rational fields

There is one further beyond-the-evidence category: we make beyond-the-evidence decisions (either knowingly or instinctively) to organise types of evidence and non-evidence in rational fields (or purposive systems).

Rational fields are fully discussed in **Part Two** of this book. With the exception of **Type 8**, the place of evidence and non-evidence in our assessments of the world can be illustrated like this (see **Figure 2**):

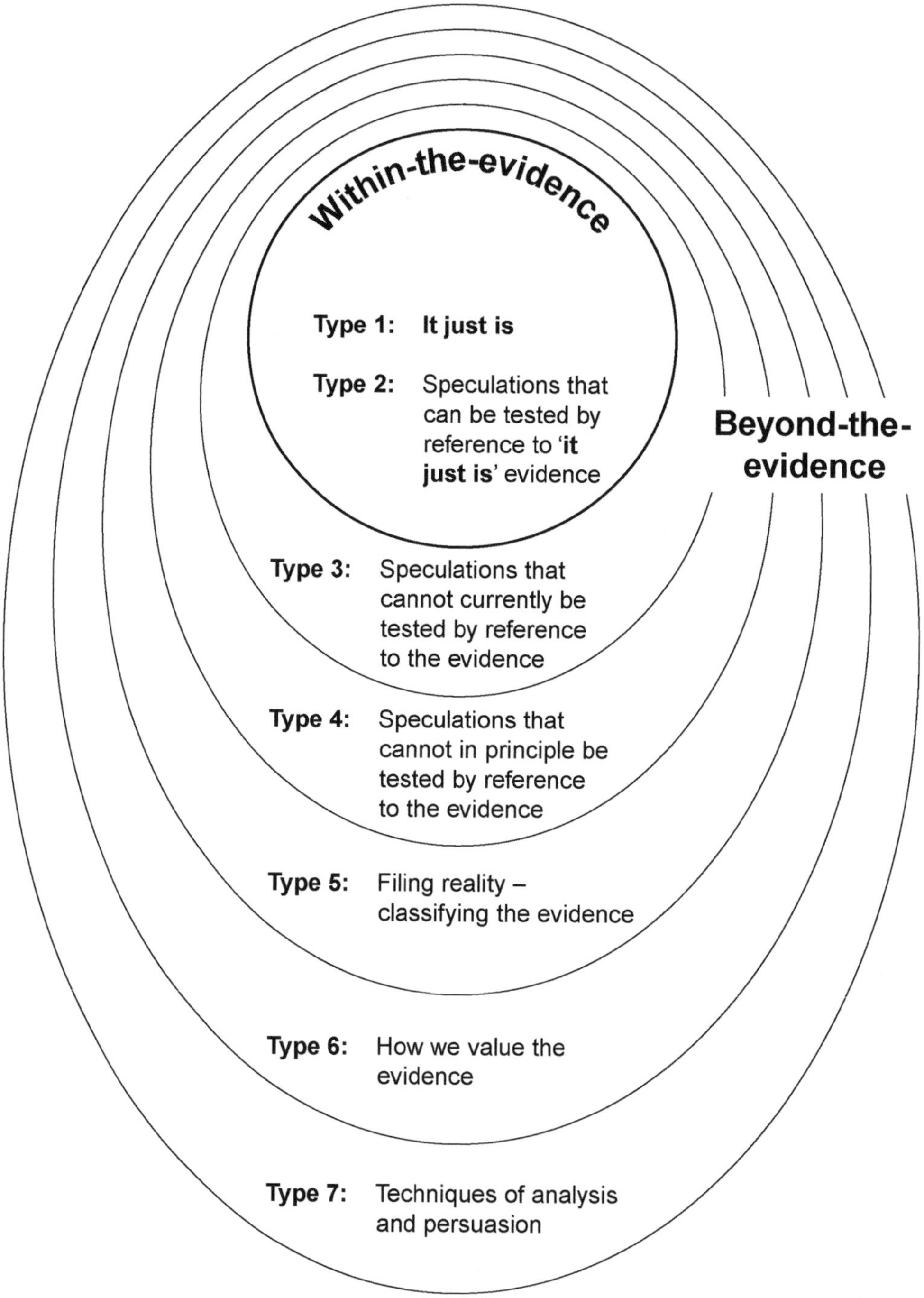
Within-the-evidence
Type 1: It just is
Type 2: Speculations that can be tested by reference to 'it just is' evidence
Beyond-the-evidence
Type 3: Speculations that cannot currently be tested by reference to the evidence
Type 4: Speculations that cannot in principle be tested by reference to the evidence
Type 5: Filing reality – classifying the evidence
Type 6: How we value the evidence
Type 7: Techniques of analysis and persuasion

Figure 2 Types of evidence and non-evidence

The urge to make sense of things

By referring to **Figure 2**, it is easy to see what was happening in the Christchurch courtroom. It's impossible for us to deal with the world without reasons. We need explanations. We need diagnoses. We need labels. We need to translate the evidence into a form we can cope with. And as we rush to make sense of things we assume that of all the different ways of interpreting the evidence, one of them must be right. Consequently, we tend to look for parcelled-up answers: the girls had abnormal brains, they were mentally ill, they were legally insane, they were wild-cats, they had antisocial natures, they were sexually insatiable, they were evil, they were possessed. Once we hit on an answer that satisfies us, we feel better: that's why they did it, now we know.

But we don't really know. Most of the time we are guessing or merely hoping that we've hit on it. But is it really plausible that there was a single reason for the murder? Certainly neither criminality nor insanity are useful as anything other than psychological props. To define the girls as criminal says nothing more than 'we don't approve of cold-blooded killing', and so we choose to define this sort of killing as being outside acceptable ethical and legal limits. And to designate them insane tells us only that sane people – like psychiatrists, judges and journalists? – were unable to comprehend their actions.

Alternative speculations from beyond-the-evidence

The above analysis leads to a potentially uncomfortable conclusion – that there is no difference between the four explanations of Pauline's and Juliet's thoughts and actions below:

A. The girls were possessed
B. The girls were evil
C. The girls were criminal
D. The girls were insane

A. The girls were possessed

Perhaps some supernatural force compelled the girls to do what they did. Gurr and Cox certainly believed some mysterious power took a hand:

> 'The brick crashed on her mother's head, and she collapsed. And that was the moment when Pauline wished it hadn't happened. **But some force possessed her, drove her on, some inner voice which commanded: It is too late to stop!** She struck again, and again, and now Juliet, panting from a sprint along the track, was kneeling beside her, and swinging the sling-shot.'[1] (Bold mine)

Gurr and Cox were not alone at the time, and would not be alone now. Indeed, according to a Gallup poll of a randomly selected sample of 1012 adults in the US, no fewer than 41% of Americans believe that 'people on this earth are sometimes possessed by the devil'.[14]

A fascinating religious website reports:[15]

> **Conservative Protestant beliefs and practices about exorcism**:
> Fundamentalists and other Evangelical Christians exhibit a wide range of beliefs concerning demon possession and exorcism. But most share certain fundamentals:
>
> Like Roman Catholics, most believe that the passages about demons in the New Testament are accurate descriptions of the power and activity of evil spirits.
>
> Satan and his demons are believed to be living entities who roam around the world looking for people to torment and destroy.
>
> Many view Satanic forces as playing a major role in individuals' lives today. Books in Christian bookstores and programs on Christian radio and TV frequently refer to demonic influences, and warn believers to be continuously on guard.

The site contains a fair bit of small print (quoted below as it appears at the website):

> **Some Evangelical beliefs**:
> J. F. Cogan has written a 'Demon Possession Handbook for Human Service Workser' [sic]. It is a very complete presentation of demon possession and exorcism... The handbook is intended to acquaint case workers, church workers, correction officers and 22 other professions with what he feels is the reality of demon possession. He comments: '... Satan and his demons have real power. Within the limits God has set, Satan and his demons can do real spiritual damage to humans who are not filled by and, therefore, protected by the power of the Holy Spirit.'
>
> He cites a number of behaviors and activities that are commonly caused by demon possession today:
>
> '... all serial killers and serial arsonists are demon possessed.'
>
> Intermittent demon possession is a cause of spousal abuse.
>
> 'Suicide is frequently associated with demon possession.'
>
> 'When two people are both demon possessed, they may have a lustful affinity for each other which defies all logic... Often, demon-induced lust leads to murder...'
>
> Irrational shoplifting.
>
> Childhood learning disabilities and behavioral problems.
>
> Various physical illnesses.
>
> Mental illnesses such as schizophrenia.
>
> Post-hypnotic suggestion.
>
> Demons possess houses as well as humans; a haunted house may be a 'nesting place' of evil spirits.
>
> Certain games can lead to demonic involvement: Ouija boards, dungeons and dragons and other role playing games, games involving dragons, etc.
>
> Multiple Personality Disorder (a.k.a. Dissociative Identity Disorder).
>
> False memories can be implanted by demons in the mind of a person undergoing recovered memory therapy.
>
> Spontaneous Human Combustion.
>
> Foul and abusive language in a voice that is different from the victim's normal voice.

He writes that there are many activities that can actively draw demons to the individual(s) involved:

> Illicit sex.
> Homosexual sex.
> Viewing pornography.
> Using mind-altering drugs.
> Hypnosis.
> Listening to rock music, particularly if the musicians are themselves involved with demons ...[15]

In my opinion, Mr Cogan has a pathetic outlook on the world. He looks around, sees a lot of 'very bad stuff' going on and can cope with it only by calling it the work of the devil, rather than accepting it as part of the human condition. But however much I despair of Mr Cogan's philosophy of life, I cannot defeat his opinion with an opinion of my own.

According to his view of the world (based on **Type 4** and **5** judgements) the girls were possessed by a demon. In my opinion (also based on **Type 4** and **5** judgements) the girls responded in an unusual yet perfectly rational way to a claustrophobic world that tried far too zealously to cage their independent natures. They weren't possessed and they weren't insane – they were rational creatures, trapped in God-fearing New Zealand in 1954. But I can't prove I'm right and I can't prove Mr Cogan wrong. I can point to patterns in the evidence. I can indicate logical fallacies in his reasoning. I can point out that there seems to be no evidential basis whatsoever for his beliefs – while there is a lot of support for mine. I can argue that psychotherapy works better than exorcism. I can come up with all sorts of reasoned positions, but I cannot finally overrule his beyond-the-evidence interpretation with my own.

However, the point is not whether Mr Cogan is right or I am. What is important is that we recognise that our assumptions are *essentially of the same type* as the assumptions held by those who believe in psychiatry.

B. The girls were evil

Is the world made up of good and evil? The President of the United States of America and much of the US media are convinced it is:

> Civilized people around the world denounce the evildoers who devised and executed these terrible attacks. Justice demands that those who helped or harbored the terrorists be punished – and punished severely. The enormity of their evil demands it. We will use all the resources of the United States and our cooperating friends and allies to pursue those responsible for this evil until justice is done.[16]

Were the girls evil? Dr Medlicott (one of the psychiatrists for the defence) seems to have thought so:

> 'There was,' he said, 'a gross reversal of moral sense.' **They admired those things which are evil and condemned those things the community considers good**. They had weird ideas and their own paradise, god and religion.'[3] (Bold mine)

Furthermore:

> When Mr Justice Adams passed sentence, a man in the public gallery called 'I protest!' An Australian editorial writer heard in the minds of thousands of others an echo of this cry

> against the sentence, but for a different reason: **'It is that two young human beings should ever be in such a way the victims of a dark conspiracy of circumstance so evil in its purpose and so appalling in its outcome.'**[1] (Bold mine)

On this latter view, evil is seen as an entity in itself, relentlessly stalking the girls in order to manifest its presence in the human world. But we will never know for sure whether evil really haunts the world, nor whether Pauline and Juliet were evil creatures, because the judgement that something is or is not evil rests permanently beyond-the-evidence (it is a judgement based on **Types 4, 5** and **6**).

C. The girls were criminal

Whether or not someone is regarded as a criminal depends on a human choice to establish laws defining crime. Crime in Islamic law is not the same as crime in US law. Furthermore, what counts as a specific crime, under either jurisdiction, is itself often a matter of interpretation (Did this person *truly* offend a basic Islamic principle? Did this person *recklessly* cause the death of another, or was it just carelessness?).

D. The girls were insane

> That the two girls killed Mrs. Parker was not disputed, and the jury was left mainly to decide between the Crown's submission that **the girls were sane** and the defence that **the girls were grossly insane**, and were suffering from paranoia of the exalted type in a setting of *folie à deux*.[17] (Bold mine)

It is impossible to tell which of these views is correct because – as with the other three explanations – possession, evilness and criminality – the idea of insanity exists only beyond-the-evidence.

And the same is true of any other classifications contained in psychiatric diagnostic manuals – yes there are patterns of human behaviour, yes it is plausible to group these into syndromes, yes the majority of psychiatrists can agree to call one syndrome or another by the same name. But that is by the way. In the absence of indisputable evidence that there are mental illness-causing entities and processes, everything boils down to beyond-the-evidence assumptions and decisions (see **Figure 3**).

CONCLUSION

Each supposition – possession, evilness, insanity, criminality, failed rationality – takes hard evidence (the hitting, the planning, the events) and interprets it according to an ultimately unprovable view of the world. The psychiatric view of the world is no different from any of the others, because there are indispensable beyond-the-evidence elements involved in calling something or someone ill or diseased.

The ethical import of this is huge and should be obvious: the consequences for the girls – indeed for all of us – may be very different dependent upon the classification scheme chosen from beyond-the-evidence. And since it is we – not the unadorned evidence – who choose these types of classification, we must surely examine ourselves and our reasons for choosing as we do.

This is the purpose of the rest of this book.

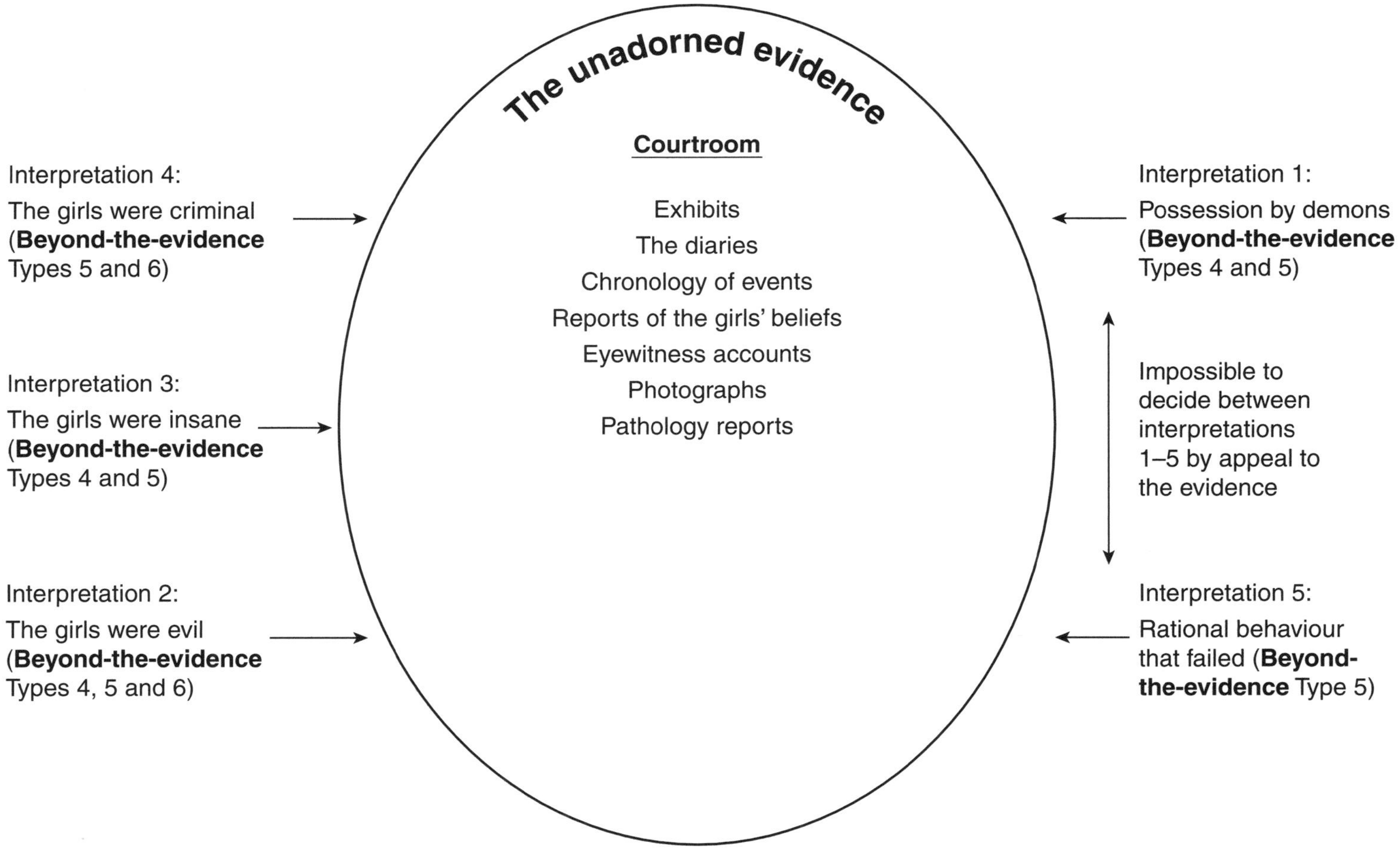
The unadorned evidence
Courtroom
Exhibits
The diaries
Chronology of events
Reports of the girls' beliefs
Eyewitness accounts
Photographs
Pathology reports
Interpretation 4:
The girls were criminal (Beyond-the-evidence Types 5 and 6)
Interpretation 3:
The girls were insane (Beyond-the-evidence Types 4 and 5)
Interpretation 2:
The girls were evil (Beyond-the-evidence Types 4, 5 and 6)
Interpretation 1:
Possession by demons (Beyond-the-evidence Types 4 and 5)
Impossible to decide between interpretations 1–5 by appeal to the evidence
Interpretation 5:
Rational behaviour that failed (Beyond-the-evidence Type 5)

Figure 3 A simplified picture of five beyond-the-evidence interpretations in the Heavenly Creatures case

POSTSCRIPT: WHAT HAPPENED TO THE HEAVENLY CREATURES?

> *Teenagers sentenced to detention for murder.* Pauline Yvonne Parker, aged 16, and Juliet Marion Hulme, aged 15 years 10 months, were sentenced in the Supreme Court on Saturday afternoon to be detained during Her Majesty's pleasure. They had just been found guilty by a jury on a charge of murdering Parker's mother, Honora Mary Parker, at Victoria Park on Tuesday, June 22. In returning their finding that the girls were guilty, the jury rejected a plea by the defence that the girls were not guilty on the grounds of insanity.[17]

Pauline and Juliet were released separately after five years. Apparently they never saw each other again. Juliet immediately went overseas. She converted to Mormonism and eventually settled in Scotland, where she changed her name to Anne Perry, and became a successful author of Victorian murder mysteries.[18] Pauline remained on probation in New Zealand, and did not leave the country until 1965. She attended Auckland University, and mixed in the Auckland lesbian community. According to a New Zealand women's magazine, she now lives as a recluse in a small English village.[19,20]

CHAPTER TWO

Psychiatry's Alchemy: An Attempt to Transform Non-Evidence Into Evidence

SUMMARY

This chapter:

- Explains that psychiatry would not exist without beyond-the-evidence assumptions
- Shows how psychiatry's faithful deceive themselves (and a lot of other people) that non-evidence is really evidence
- Concludes that alternative classifications of mental problems are equally as plausible as psychiatry's

◆

INTRODUCTION

Chapter One closed with the controversial assertion that it is impossible to use the unadorned evidence to decide between the boxed hypotheses below, because each draws on exactly the same evidence in support of its case:

> **A. The girls were possessed**
> **B. The girls were evil**
> **C. The girls were criminal**
> **D. The girls were insane**

This conclusion is controversial because to most conventionally educated Westerners, demonic possession and evilness are plainly more speculative than psychiatric explanations of strange behaviour (even given the US Gallup Poll evidence reported in Chapter One). Nevertheless, we are deceived. The psychiatric view of the world is based just as much in non-evidence as any of the alternatives.

This may look like a problem. But it is only a problem if you are convinced that the psychiatric view of the world is true. It is not a problem if you have an open mind.

This chapter explodes the myth (a straw-man, really) that psychiatry is based on rigorously scientific evidence, and is therefore a view of the human world to which we must all adhere for evermore. But it is not an anti-psychiatry tirade (there are plenty of these in circulation already). Rather the main point of the chapter is simply to bolster the argument that we don't have to stick with current health work classifications if they are not serving us well.

PSYCHIATRY: WHAT'S THE EVIDENCE AND WHAT'S BEYOND-THE-EVIDENCE?

Here are some apparent facts and figures about mental illness:

FACTS AND FIGURES ABOUT MENTAL ILLNESS

> Mental illnesses are health conditions characterized by alterations in thinking, mood, or behavior (or some combination) associated with distress and/or impaired functioning.
>
> i Of American adults, 5.4 percent have a serious mental illness (SMI).[21]
>
> (*Note – An individual is said to have a severe mental illness (SMI) when he or she meets the criteria for a DSM disorder during a 12-month period (excluding substance use disorders and developmental disorders) causing functional impairment. Functional impairment is defined as substantial interference with one or more major life activities including basic daily living skills (e.g., eating and bathing), instrumental living skills (e.g., maintaining a household and managing money), and functioning in social, family, and vocational/educational contexts.)
>
> ii Twenty-three percent of American adults (ages 18 and older) suffer from a diagnosable mental disorder in a given year, but only half report impairment of their daily functioning due to the mental disorder. Six percent of adults have addictive disorders alone, and three percent have both mental and addictive disorders.[22]
>
> iii Almost half of the adults with serious and persistent mental illnesses are between the ages of 25 and 44.[23]
>
> iv Approximately nine percent to 13 percent of children ages nine to 17 have a serious emotional disturbance with substantial functional impairment, and five percent to nine percent have a serious emotional disturbance with extreme functional impairment due to a mental illness ...[24]
>
> vi Four of the ten leading causes of disability in the United States and other developed countries are mental disorders, which include major depression, bipolar disorder, schizophrenia, and obsessive-compulsive disorder ...[21]

> ix The total cost of mental health services in the U.S. was $148 billion in 1990. The direct cost of mental health services (treatment and rehabilitation costs) totaled $69 billion, and the indirect costs (lost productivity at work, school, or home due to disability or death) were estimated at $78.6 billion...[25]
>
> xiii In 1998, 283,800 people with mental illnesses were incarcerated in American prisons and jails. This is four times the number of people in state mental hospitals throughout the country.[26,27]

On the face of it this is staggering. According to the National Alliance for the Mentally Ill (**NAMI**) (a pro-psychiatry parents' movement which believes that mental illnesses are brain-related disorders) a quarter of American adults have a mental disorder. Indeed, according to **NAMI**'s figures, well over a third of young US adults are mentally ill, since the prevalence of mental disorder is higher among younger people. Furthermore, a fifth of American children are seriously mentally ill and mental health services cost well over a hundred billion dollars annually. Mental illness appears to be a frightening epidemic, just about out of control.

Fortunately (perhaps) help is at hand from scientists, psychiatrists and socially-concerned drug companies:

> Mental illnesses are disorders of the brain that disrupt a person's thinking, feeling, moods, and ability to relate to others. Just as diabetes is a disorder of the pancreas, mental illnesses are brain disorders that often result in a diminished capacity for coping with the ordinary demands of life...
>
> ...Most importantly, these brain disorders are treatable. As a diabetic takes insulin, most people with serious mental illness need medication to help control symptoms.[27]

According to the school of thought that all mental illness is biologically based, schizophrenia is the most prevalent of the mental illnesses:

> At any given time, between 1 percent and 2 percent of the world's population – including 1 to 2 million American adults – is afflicted with schizophrenia. It is the single most destructive disease to young lives. Men and women are at equal risk of developing this illness; however, most males become ill between 16 and 25 years old; females develop symptoms between ages 25 and 30.
>
> Conventional antipsychotic drugs, such as haloperidol, chlorpromazine, and fluphenazine have been available since the mid-1950s. These drugs primarily block dopamine receptors and are effective in treating the 'positive' symptoms of schizophrenia.
>
> The newer antipsychotics, serotonin-dopamine antagonists (SDAs) block both serotonin and dopamine receptors, thereby treating both the 'positive' and 'negative' symptoms of schizophrenia.[28]

(Readers should note that this quote is taken from a website maintained by the Janssen Pharmaceutical Research Foundation.)

According to the biopsychiatrists, the evidence is unequivocal:

> Years of research have shown that schizophrenia is a biologically based brain disease. The most recent advances in brain imaging have confirmed imbalances of two brain chemicals – dopamine and serotonin – in those who suffer from schizophrenia. Dopamine is responsible for emotions and motivation; serotonin acts as a messenger and stimulates muscle movement, switching nerves on and off. The brains of people with schizophrenia have elevated dopamine and serotonin activity.[28]

This mixture of assertion and statistic is presented so often by psychiatry and its supporters that it has become 'public knowledge':

> What the profession communicates to the public through the media is summed up in a recent newspaper headline: GENETIC BASIS OF SCHIZOPHRENIA SAID TO BE FOUND.
>
> Books written for lay-people also make the claim that the hereditary basis of madness is a fact rather than a bias or conjecture... assertions of this kind are so frequent that even sophisticated scientists in other fields assume that schizophrenia must have a proven genetic link.
>
> Similarly a constant stream of propaganda from psychiatry tells the public that all forms of human distress are due to biochemical imbalances or even gross brain damage.[29]

Everyone knows that psychiatrists use drugs and electro-shock to treat mental illness, so most of us assume that mental illness must be caused by the brain problems the drugs and electricity attack. However, like all views about mental illness and mental health, these apparent certainties depend on beyond-the-evidence assumptions. As always, the evidence does not speak for itself.

Peter Breggin, a leading critic of modern psychiatry, and a psychiatrist himself, is part of an anti-psychiatry movement that challenges what he calls 'misleading psychiatric slogans'. Anti-psychiatrists argue that though it is possible to dull the symptoms of schizophrenia using drugs or surgery, this does not mean that the parts of the brain affected are the primary cause of the symptoms. If you unplug a TV set you get rid of the pictures – but the TV set itself is not the essential cause of the pictures, it is just what they run on. Equally, the brain is not necessarily the cause of overwhelming thoughts – the thoughts need the brain just as a TV programme needs a TV, but they are not caused by the brain alone. Both TV programmes and human thoughts are created by a complicated interplay of meaning, purpose, and social and intellectual experience. In other words, it **just is** the case – **Type 1** – that drugs and surgery do what they do, but the conclusion that mental illness is therefore a brain problem remains a **Type 3** speculation.

Breggin is especially critical of psychiatry's perpetual assumption that its hypotheses (almost all of which are of **Type 3** and beyond) are, or follow from, **Type 1** or **2** evidence:

> The most frequently cited possible cause of schizophrenia is an abnormal hyperactivity of the dopamine transmitter system in the brain... What is the theory? In a nutshell, since the neuroleptics probably achieve their effect on schizophrenic patients primarily by suppressing dopamine nerve transmission, we may speculate that dopamine neurotransmitters are abnormally hyperactive in schizophrenics.
>
> The neuroleptics do suppress dopamine activity in various parts of the higher brain, including the main nerve pathways to the frontal lobes and emotion regulating limbic system... closely related to the ones that are cut in psychosurgery...
>
> Because the neuroleptics inhibit dopamine nerve transmission in the frontal lobes, should we suppose there's something wrong with these areas of the brain? Not at all... these drugs have the same effect on all people, regardless of their diagnosis or mental condition. They always inhibit passion and willpower. They even have this effect on animals...
>
> Consider alcohol and its impact on us. For many people, alcohol provides at least a brief sense of relaxation, and maybe even euphoria. Alcohol accomplishes this by impeding brain function, and, with chronic use, it disables brain cells and can kill them. Does this

mean there is something wrong with these brain cells because people 'feel better' when the cells are disabled or even dead?

...there's no way to prove the hyperactive dopamine hypothesis at present, because the studies are almost always done on patients who have taken neuroleptic drugs.[30]

AN ANTIDOTE TO ALCHEMY

Establishing what is within-the-evidence and what is beyond can be refreshingly clarifying in the pro- *versus* anti-psychiatry debate. To this end revisit **Figure 2**, the relevant parts of which are listed below:

WITHIN-THE-EVIDENCE

Type 1: It just is
Type 2: Testable speculations

BEYOND-THE-EVIDENCE

Type 3: Speculations that cannot currently be tested
Type 4: Speculations that cannot in principle be tested
Type 5: Ways of filing reality
Type 6: Valuing evidence

By using these **Types** it is possible to disentangle the merits of the various claims and counter-claims made in the voluminous literature. For example, there is much that **just is** the case. It **just is** the case that all sorts of brain abnormalities and injury can affect thinking and action. There is no doubt about this – people's intellectual, emotional and cognitive capacities can change radically as a result of injury, malfunction (a 'stroke' for example) and indeed medication (many people treated with anti-psychotic medication report that their very personality changes as the drugs take effect).[31] It also **just is** the case that certain areas of the brain are associated with certain types of thinking and behaviour – we have technologies (brain scans, for example) and associated theories that produce evidence with which we can test our **Type 2** speculations.

However, it is equally clear that brain malfunction – chemical, physical or electrical – is by no means the whole story of why things go well or badly for people with brain abnormalities. Factors such as our approval or disapproval of behaviours (**Types 5** and **6**), social expectations (**Types 5** and **6**), levels of protection and support for the person with the abnormality (**Type 6**), the way statistically normal people view people who think differently (**Type 5**), and much else, also play a part.

THE WHAT TYPE OF EVIDENCE TEST

The **what type of evidence test** is very simple. It merely takes claims about the status of evidence, and classifies them according to the six **Types** listed above and illustrated in **Figure 2**. Below, it is applied to a recent summary of the state of contemporary psychiatry written by a widely respected scientist of psychiatry, and also to some comments from anti-psychiatry critics. The topic of the summary is schizophrenia. However, many of the article's points are commonly used in defence of biopsychiatry in general.

PROGRESS IN PSYCHIATRY: THE OFFICIAL VIEW

This summary of biopsychiatric thinking about the causes and treatment of schizophrenia appeared as an editorial in the prestigious US medical journal, the *New England Journal of Medicine*.[32] It is presented here in an abbreviated form.

The editorial is worth careful inspection, much more for what it reveals about how much is *not* known and how much is speculation than for its account of within-the-evidence progress in psychiatry. Its author, Nancy Andreasen (who also helped formulate the *American Psychiatric Association's* (APA) diagnostic rule-book, the DSM-III[33]) begins:

> Schizophrenia is one of our most important public health problems. It is a common, tragic, and devastating mental illness that typically strikes young people just when they are maturing into adulthood.

A common feature of writing about mental illness by both pro- and anti-psychiatry authors is the tendency to assume the truth of explanations that fit with other explanations they accept already. In the extract above, Andreasen first assumes that there is an illness or disease (it is unclear which) called schizophrenia. This is both a **Type 5** decision (to file a range of symptoms under the heading schizophrenia) and, for reasons Andreasen herself outlines in the bulk of her article, it is also a **Type 3** speculation that cannot currently be tested. Andreasen then takes **Type 1 'just is'** evidence that adolescents often find maturing into adulthood so difficult they experience delusions (evidence which may have nothing whatsoever to do with schizophrenia) and she attempts alchemy. Hey presto, the 'fact' that adolescents are especially affected by 'schizophrenia' instantly becomes yet further proof that schizophrenia exists.

Andreasen does not mean to commit a deception – rather she is deceived herself.[34] She is deceived because she has confused the psychiatric filing system with **just is** reality. She believes the filing cabinet sits within-the-evidence. But it does not – as anyone not ideologically committed to the belief that 'schizophrenia exists' can see.

There are several alternative interpretations of the **Type 1** evidence that young people find it hard to grow out of 'adolescence' (itself a **Type 5** category). Peter Breggin writes:

> People undergoing spiritual crisis – romantic love, adolescence... – are frequently rebellious and sometimes revolutionary. They commonly find themselves in conflict

> with one or another authority, from parents and police to religious and educational institutions. This happens because they frequently tend to put their immediate spiritual needs and priorities above the demands of authority, and because they often handle their conflicts with authority in an ineffective, self-defeating or helpless manner...
>
> Where passionate, spirited encounters with the meaning of life take place, ordinary concepts of responsibility often get left behind. Sometimes it seems as if people must temporarily reject or throw off responsibility in the process of reaching new plateaus. That they become exceedingly difficult to live with does not make them 'mentally ill' or diseased...
>
> People are often labelled schizophrenic during their teen years. Adolescence, with its struggle to form identity in the face of unleashed passions, easily gets called 'mental illness'. Whether adolescents become labelled mentally ill often depends mostly on the love, patience and tolerance of the adults who surround them.
>
> After passionate people get psychiatrically labelled, they become especially vulnerable to defeat and disaster. Psychiatrists commonly force treatment upon them, then claim that they must be 'mentally ill' because they resent and resist being diagnosed and treated.[35]

Schizophrenia is only one of many possible ways of classifying young people's battles to adapt to the adult world. Perhaps it is true that the brains of troubled youngsters are diseased. Or perhaps adolescents look at the adult world, and the adult world looks crazy. Who wants a mortgage, a job and a pension plan when there are all these places to explore and questions to ask – like, 'Why am I alive?' 'Who am I?' and 'What am I going to do in this terrifying place?' But the adolescent is inexorably trapped by pervasive adult conventions, lack of experience and (usually) lack of money. When he or she responds in desperate ways, perhaps the diagnosis of schizophrenia is nothing more than a defensive response of pompous adults who have forgotten their own adolescence. Certainly, a diagnosis of schizophrenia not only tends to remove at least some blame from the adolescent, it also deflects attention from parents and a social system obsessed with dress, money, glamour and fame.

Of course, this non-psychiatric interpretation is beyond-the-evidence too – it is either **Type 3** or **4**; it is definitely **Type 5** and stems from **Type 6** values. But this merely means that both views – pro- and non-psychiatric – stem equally from beyond-the-evidence. So why should the psychiatric view be so dominant?

It should also be remembered that even if a biological cause of some kind could be established beyond doubt – even if the idea that 'schizophrenia exists' could be shown to be of **Type 2** – a multitude of beyond-the-evidence judgements would remain. These would include, for example, the belief that biological abnormality or damage is a problem (leucotomy is brain damage but it wasn't seen as a problem by the surgeons who routinely performed leucotomies throughout several twentieth-century decades), the notion that children killing parents is a problem (it isn't in all cultures), the idea that certain behaviours are evidence of a sickness, the view that mentally sick people are not responsible for their actions, and so on.

THE EMPTY SCHIZOPHRENIA HYPOTHESIS

Just like the medieval alchemists, psychiatry's apparent strength is its claim to be a science, or at least to be based on science. But a simple review of the 'schizophrenia hypothesis' – as advanced by one of psychiatry's most prominent advocates – quickly and fatally undermines it.

Andreasen writes that:

> Both its (schizophrenia's) symptoms and signs and its associated cognitive abnormalities are too diverse to permit its localization in a single region of the brain.[32]

This confession ought to give schizophrenia's advocates significant pause for thought, at the very least. Biopsychiatry says that schizophrenia is a disease of the brain (a **Type 5** assumption advertised as **Type 1**). Yet unlike brain diseases that have an exact location and so really **just are** (abnormal cell growth, for instance) the place where the 'schizophrenia disease' resides is unknown. And not only is the location of schizophrenia a mystery, but its very nature is 'diverse' too.

This leaves schizophrenia as nothing more precise than a complex and widespread set of thoughts and behaviours whose seat in the brain is unknown. Or, in Andreasen's words:

> The working hypothesis shared by most investigators is that schizophrenia is a disease of neural connectivity caused by multiple factors that affect brain development.[36] (and see refs 37 and 34)

The nature of hypotheses is that they may or may not be correct, but working psychiatrists and psychiatric scientists routinely assume that the 'schizophrenia is a disease' hypothesis is true (making a **Type 5** guess). Yet instead of the certainty about schizophrenia so confidently proclaimed by those who have worldly reason to believe in it, in truth we have nothing more than speculation.

> Our current model of the causation of schizophrenia is very similar to that used to understand cancer. That is, schizophrenia probably occurs as a consequence of multiple 'hits,' which include **some combination** of inherited genetic factors and external, nongenetic factors that affect the regulation and expression of genes governing brain function or that injure the brain directly. Some people may have a genetic predisposition that requires a convergence of additional factors to produce the expression of the disorder. This convergence results in abnormalities in brain development and maturation, a process that is ongoing during the first two decades of life.[38] The abnormalities are typically not focal but, rather, involve distributed neural circuits and neurotransmitter systems.[32] (Bold mine)

What this 'some combination' is, is not known. Believe it or not, this means that the 'schizophrenia hypothesis' is merely: *many factors in brains cause an unlocalised brain disease which has diverse symptoms and signs.*

This hypothesis says nothing, and can tell us nothing. It is not even **Type 3**. It is **Type 4**.

For illustration, here are some parallel **Type 4** hypotheses:

> *Many factors in tomato plants cause an unlocalised tomato plant disease which has diverse symptoms and signs*
>
> *Many factors in children cause an unlocalised children's disease which has diverse symptoms and signs*
>
> *Many factors in cognition cause an unlocalised cognitive disease which has diverse symptoms and signs*

These are useless hypotheses too. They cannot be tested by the evidence, even in principle, since everything seems to confirm them (any of the diverse symptoms can be said to be caused by any of the multiple factors in any combination) and nothing can possibly refute them.[39]

Andreasen assumes that all the factors and symptoms in 'schizophrenia' are ultimately connected:

> When the connectivity and communication within neural circuitry are disrupted, patients have a variety of symptoms and impairments in cognition. Behind this diversity, however, is a final common pathway that defines the illness. For schizophrenia, it is misregulation of information processing in the brain. Ongoing etiologic studies must focus on finding the origins of abnormalities that lie beneath the clinical surface.
>
> These symptoms and signs occur in patterns that may not overlap; one patient may have hallucinations and affective flattening, whereas another has disorganized speech and avolition. The diversity and nonoverlapping pattern of symptoms and signs suggest a more basic and unifying problem: abnormalities in neural circuits and fundamental cognitive mechanisms.[40] (and see ref. 41)

But why look for a 'final common pathway'? Since schizophrenia is simply an hypothesis, and '... the symptoms and signs of schizophrenia are (so) diverse... they encompass the entire range of human mental activity...', then the thought that there might be a 'final common pathway' is merely another hypothesis – and a wildly speculative one to anyone not indoctrinated in medicine's ubiquitous faith in 'final common pathways'.

In the world outside biopsychiatry's filing cabinet, such a multiplicity of phenomena would strongly suggest that there is *no* common cause – and no final common pathway to be found. If I were to discover that the various species of plants in my garden were all suffering from black blotches I would feel entitled to hypothesise that there was a common cause. Yet if I were to find that the plants were suffering from a multiplicity of unwanted phenomena – bugs, dropping leaves, mould, rotten stems, no fruit, red spots, and so on – then it would, I think, be astonishingly stupid of me to assume a single cause.

> Patients with schizophrenia also have impairment in many different cognitive systems, such as memory, attention, and executive function. This is often referred to as a generalized deficit, and its existence provides additional support for the likelihood that the disorder is the result of a basic process such as a general impairment in the coordination of information processing.[40] (and see ref. 41)

The notion that 'generalized deficit' is the result of 'general impairment' looks like desperation, just as it would if I explained my gardening problems in the same way.

Indeed, abandon the assumption that schizophrenia is a disease and an apparent cause can instantly become an effect:

> **The Chicken and the Egg**
> Suppose future studies of schizophrenic patients do document a relative degree of dopamine hyperactivity in all or some of them. Would this prove that these people's brains are abnormal or that dopamine causes the schizophrenia? Commonsense and experimental evidence indicates that certain passionate states are associated with corresponding changes in brain function. Prolonged mental stresses of almost any kind, as well as physical trauma or stress, cause the brain to stimulate increased production of certain hormones, such as steroids. Conversely, if you are relaxing right now, your steroid

output may decline. In each of these instances the mental state influenced the brain, rather than vice versa...

...a whole new field is developing, psychoimmunology, based on the theory that our state of mind affects our brain, which in turn affects our immunological system.

Clearly, proving an association between a particular state of mind and a particular reaction in the brain doesn't indicate which came first. Yet the biopsychiatrists, without discussing it, usually assume that the brain is the egg from which the chicken – mental disorder – is born. They search for signs of hyperactivity in the dopamine system of schizophrenics without acknowledging that if they find it, it could be the *normal* response of a *normal brain* to the prolonged expression of an intense emotional state.[42]

Because the schizophrenia hypothesis is so vague, further speculations about schizophrenia's causes are given free rein in the psychiatric literature. Andreasen gives some examples:

As discussed by Mortensen et al. in this issue of the Journal,[43] schizophrenia runs in families, and twin and adoption studies indicate that such familial aggregation is largely accounted for by genetic factors. However, the same studies also indicate that familial genetic transmission can account for only a portion of the cases of schizophrenia; for example, the concordance rate in monozygotic twins is approximately 40 percent, suggesting that nongenetic factors must also have a role. Genetically, schizophrenia resembles other complex illnesses, such as diabetes mellitus, in that it is nonmendelian, probably polygenic, and probably multifactorial. Recent linkage, association, and candidate-gene studies suggest multiple susceptibility loci, including some on chromosomes 6, 8, and 22.[44]

As always, there are contrary (**Type 3**) hypotheses, and as yet we have no means of telling which, if any, are correct:

Schizophrenia does tend to run in families. About one in ten families with a schizophrenic parent will have schizophrenic offspring... [but]... [f]amilies share both a genetic and an environmental influence... share political outlooks, national feelings, cultural values and prejudices, and language...

The Meaning of Twin Studies
Identical twins have shown a tendency toward concordance for schizophrenia... but usually less than half the time.

Can we think of any good reasons, other than genetics, why madness might sometimes afflict both members of a pair of identical twins? Indeed, wouldn't we *expect* it to happen sometimes as a result of the similarity of their environments as children? Especially in the decades in which these studies were done, parents typically tried to rear twins with a rigorous sameness, right down to their clothing...

[In] *Not in Our Genes* (1984), R. C. Lewontin, Steven Rose, and Leon Kamin question the methodology of the twin studies, including whether the twins were really identical and whether their diagnoses were reliable. The authors confirm that in most instances, when one identical twin becomes schizophrenic, the other does not (and that)... the twin data is [sic] more compatible with an environmental influence than a genetic one.[45]

Andreasen and other biopsychiatrists acknowledge this possibility – but this only heightens their speculative enthusiasm:

Not only are multiple genes probably involved, but the nongenetic factors are likely to be multiple as well, as demonstrated by the study by Mortensen et al.[43] They found that both a family history of schizophrenia and nongenetic factors, such as birth during the winter and birth in an urban area, increased the relative risk of schizophrenia. These findings highlight the probability that the clinical manifestations of schizophrenia result from an

> unfortunate convergence of interacting causal factors. Their results suggest that infections during pregnancy or childhood and other factors related to urban birth may play a part in causing schizophrenia. Other possible nongenetic factors contributing to increased risk include the effects of poor nutrition on fetal and childhood brain development, exposure to toxins that damage neurons or affect neurotransmitter systems (e.g., alcohol, amphetamines, and retinoids), and exposure to radiation that might induce mutations.[44]

Dates of hospital admission and dates of birth of schizophrenics,[46] and evidence linking lifelong neurological problems to schizophrenia have also been suggested in the never-ending drip-drip of biopsychiatry literature. The latter hunch is based on the fact that at six months about a third of babies are two weeks or more 'late' in sitting up. One study showed that for those who later developed schizophrenia, two-thirds were late,[47] causing the researchers to draw the conclusion they wanted. A higher rate of schizophrenia was also found among children in the Netherlands born to women who were pregnant in the winter of 1944–45, when the Nazis blockaded Dutch cities.[48] According to the investigators, this suggests that malnutrition could also play a role...

But enough already, things have gotten too fantastic. On the one hand biopsychiatry tells us that problems with thinking are multifactorial, and that the picture is so complicated that it is presently impossible to establish any meaningful aetiology (virtually anything might turn out to be the key causative factor in schizophrenia). On the other hand, hundreds of individual researchers are beavering away to discover very specific causes, as if finding the magic one will provide the golden solution to all the diverse symptoms psychiatrists file under S for schizophrenia.

Of course it might be the case that:

> Since schizophrenia persists as an illness despite the fact that the majority of its victims do not marry or procreate, and since it appears to have the same lifetime prevalence throughout the world, it seems likely that multiple different, nonspecific, nongenetic factors that affect neurodevelopment are implicated.[32]

Or it might be that schizophrenia is a fiction entirely created beyond-the-evidence.

MAYBE SCHIZOPHRENIA IS A FICTION

It is interesting to reflect on Andreasen's report of the **just is** fact that:

> Unlike other mental illnesses that are also characterized by deficits in multiple cognitive systems (e.g., Alzheimer's disease), however, schizophrenia does not usually involve deterioration or progress to dementia. Instead, the degree of impairment is relatively stable after an initial fulminant course, which may last for several years. After that point, cognitive function may even improve.[49]

Under Andreasen's biopsychiatric interpretation 'schizophrenia' becomes a 'self-limiting' disease – a disease that can sometimes be 'in remission'. An alternative interpretation is that given the right support, or even left alone to work things through, people who have '... overwhelming feelings of fragmented identity, humiliation and helplessness'[50] recover, and even grow past 'schizophrenia', discovering important insights about life and themselves in the process.[51]

This pattern of people growing past supposed (**Type 5**) diseases is not only found in schizophrenia. It happens in many other 'psychiatric illnesses', including cases of 'drug addiction' and 'gambling addiction'. Peter Cohen[52] has shown that 'policy is irrelevant' to the prevention of 'drug misuse'. After a while people's lives change – they get careers, they get married, they have kids – and they no longer want to use the drugs they did. Max Abbott[53] has found a similar phenomenon in people 'addicted to gambling' – whether or not they use clinical services many 'problem gamblers' move on, overcoming their supposed addictions while still continuing to gamble.

Seen this way these problems are not diseases at all, they are stages in human development. What a tragedy it will be if it turns out that psychiatry is nothing more than unasked for interference in a natural process of spiritual growth.

WERE THE HEAVENLY CREATURES SCHIZOPHRENIC?

It would be easy enough to use the *American Psychiatric Association's* diagnostic classifications[54] to label the girls with one version of schizophrenia or another (they exhibited signs of persecution, paranoia, grandiose ideation, delusions, lack of insight into consequences, and more), and it is rather surprising that the Christchurch psychiatrists did not take this line. Whatever the case, the meaning of the girls' thoughts and behaviours is open to wide interpretation. And, as we have seen, the biopsychiatric hypothesis is no better placed than any alternative hypotheses in this regard.

CONCLUSION

What has been established so far? And what is the point of it?

Perhaps it is best to say first of all what has *not* been established. The first two chapters of this book have not shown that psychiatry is pointless, that all psychiatry is unscientific, that psychiatry's methods are ineffective, that psychiatrists are 'agents of social control', or that psychiatry is unethical. This was not the intention.

Psychiatry is a large discipline with many thousands of members. Its methods are diverse and its research is extensive. Psychiatry has developed a sophisticated taxonomy of types of illness and patterns of symptoms. The psychiatric profession has thoroughly investigated the effects of drugs and surgery on brains, bodies and thinking. And psychiatrists undeniably have the expertise to use a combination of therapies to alleviate distressing beliefs, habits and images.

All of this **just is**. However, what is not the case – and what has been directly challenged in **Chapters One** and **Two** – is the view that psychiatry enjoys a privileged interpretation of patterns of illness and effects of drugs and other therapies. Psychiatrists would have us believe that the psychiatric view of the evidence is much more certain – if not infinitely more certain – than any other view. But this is merely an attempt to transmute a favoured set of interpretations of the evidence into the only true version – and it is a deceit.

This deceit allows the profession to dominate the interpretation and treatment of mental problems to such an extent that 'psychiatry' and 'mental health' are generally thought to be synonymous. And this, in turn, means that those who are interested in mental health promotion (and in helping people cope with general life difficulties) have to fight very hard indeed to have psychiatry concede even the possibility that mental health promotion means more than 'the prevention of mental disorders'.[55]

And this is the book's main criticism of psychiatry: psychiatry's monopoly on how we should understand our lives ossifies the potential for creative solutions to life's difficulties, and it diminishes our potential for understanding ourselves and our existential travail. Psychiatry has created the belief that if you have a mental problem then you are probably mentally ill, and if you are mentally ill then the only place to get help is psychiatry – and furthermore that if you want *not* to be mentally ill or want to stay mentally healthy then psychiatrists are the only health promotion experts you need.

In a simple way, the first two chapters of this book have tried to demonstrate how easily we fall into the trap of believing that our invented classifications are real. This psychological weakness has a powerful hold on us, but there is little cogent reason to remain trapped. If psychiatry is one speculation among many, if psychiatry relies as much on beyond-the-evidence assumptions as any other speculation, why should we be bound by it? Why shouldn't we explore the alternatives openly? Why shouldn't we feel free to pick those parts of psychiatry that are helpful and combine them with other quite different autonomy-promoting options? Why shouldn't we abandon psychiatry if it isn't working for us? Why shouldn't we choose to promote health from a theoretical standpoint that has nothing to do with psychiatry, or indeed any other of the fixed views of reality we inherit from social precedent?

The health promotion field is not fixed forever. It is certainly less set than medical and legal fields. There is everything to play for, and many good reasons to reorient work for health. **Chapter Three** examines one attempt to change the direction of mental health work, from work against brain disorder to work explicitly in favour of mental health.

CHAPTER THREE

Mental Health Defined – And Disconnected

SUMMARY

This chapter:

- Outlines various definitions of mental health
- Shows that all definitions of mental health sit unmovably beyond-the-evidence
- Explains that it is therefore impossible to arbitrate between definitions of mental health within-the-evidence
- Points out that because we habitually separate 'the mental' from 'the physical', we have artificially disconnected our definitions of mental health from the physical and social world
- Argues that this disconnection is a mistaken classification of reality

WHAT IS MENTAL HEALTH?

No one can prove, by pointing to the evidence alone, that the Heavenly Creatures were mentally ill. It is equally impossible to establish that they were possessed, or evil, or even criminal on the evidence alone. And it is just as impossible to show that they – or anyone else – are now unequivocally mentally healthy. Although some aspects of evidence and theory can be tested in assertions about mental disease and brain damage, no assertion about mental health can ever be tested by direct reference to the evidence. Assertions of mental health are always and forever based in non-evidence **Types 4, 5** and **6** (see **Figure 2**).

For example, for most of us, getting on with other people is desirable. Generally speaking this makes us happy – this **just is** the case (**Type 1**). As a consequence, many people choose to call 'getting on with other people' a sign of mental health. Once this has been decided the health promotion question immediately becomes 'how can we best get on with other people?' (or, 'how can we best promote this sort of mental health?'). The answer to this question *can* be found within-the-evidence – there is an ocean of evidence to draw on to answer it. If you want to get on with people you should listen to them, express interest in them and be consistent toward them.[56,57]

Crucially, however, there is no evidence that can ever prove the assumption that getting on with people is what being mentally healthy means.

The claim that someone is mentally ill or healthy can be rendered partly testable provided beyond-the-evidence decisions to define the terms in a particular way are accepted. If someone states that mental health means 'not having brain disease' then she, and all who agree with her definition, will sometimes be able to tell if someone is mentally healthy, so long as they have the necessary equipment to detect brain disease (and so long as they agree about what counts as brain disease). However, the claim that 'mental health means not having brain disease' is not a testable assertion in the same way that 'Boyle's Law applies in all physical circumstances' is a testable assertion. Deciding that someone or some behaviour is or is not mentally healthy involves an unprovable assumption (that mental health means what it is said to mean), whereas the formula $P_1 \times V_1 = P_2 \times V_2$ applies whether we choose to call it Boyle's Law, Pressure Law or Ronald Rat's Law.[58]

The Heavenly Creatures affair perfectly illustrates the point. On casual inspection it looks obvious that the girls did not have mental health. Nevertheless, evidence that a child has killed its parent is evidence only that the killing has happened – it is not evidence that the child actually was evil or ill or unhealthy. Even in such a brutal case, whether the girls were mentally healthy or not is an open question. The Christchurch court heard that Pauline and Juliet were at times anguished, desperate and unhappy (which many people would list as features of bad mental health). And yet they were also indisputably cool, confident and strategic (markers of good mental health for most of us) (see **Figure 4**).

THINKING SERIOUSLY ABOUT MENTAL HEALTH

Powerful psychiatric associations continually claim to be 'working for mental health' (as if it is obvious to everyone that this is what they are doing) while the great majority of psychiatrists unreflectively accept that mental health is the absence of disease and illness. The serious exploration of the meaning of mental health can rattle this blind faith, and therefore we should insist on it until psychiatrists realise that they have an obligation to think properly before they act in their powerful ways. Careful thinking about how to define mental health can also highlight alternatives to the psychiatric goals of symptom control and patient and public safety.

Were mental health professionals to think honestly about the meanings of mental health, they would discover a relatively extensive literature outside their clinical textbooks. The proposals contained in these books and papers may be crudely grouped into 'conventional' and 'alternative' speculations about mental health, as illustrated in **Figure 5**.

CONVENTIONAL ACCOUNTS OF MENTAL HEALTH

According to Marie Jahoda, who extensively investigated the meaning of mental health,[59] the three most common definitions of mental health are the absence of

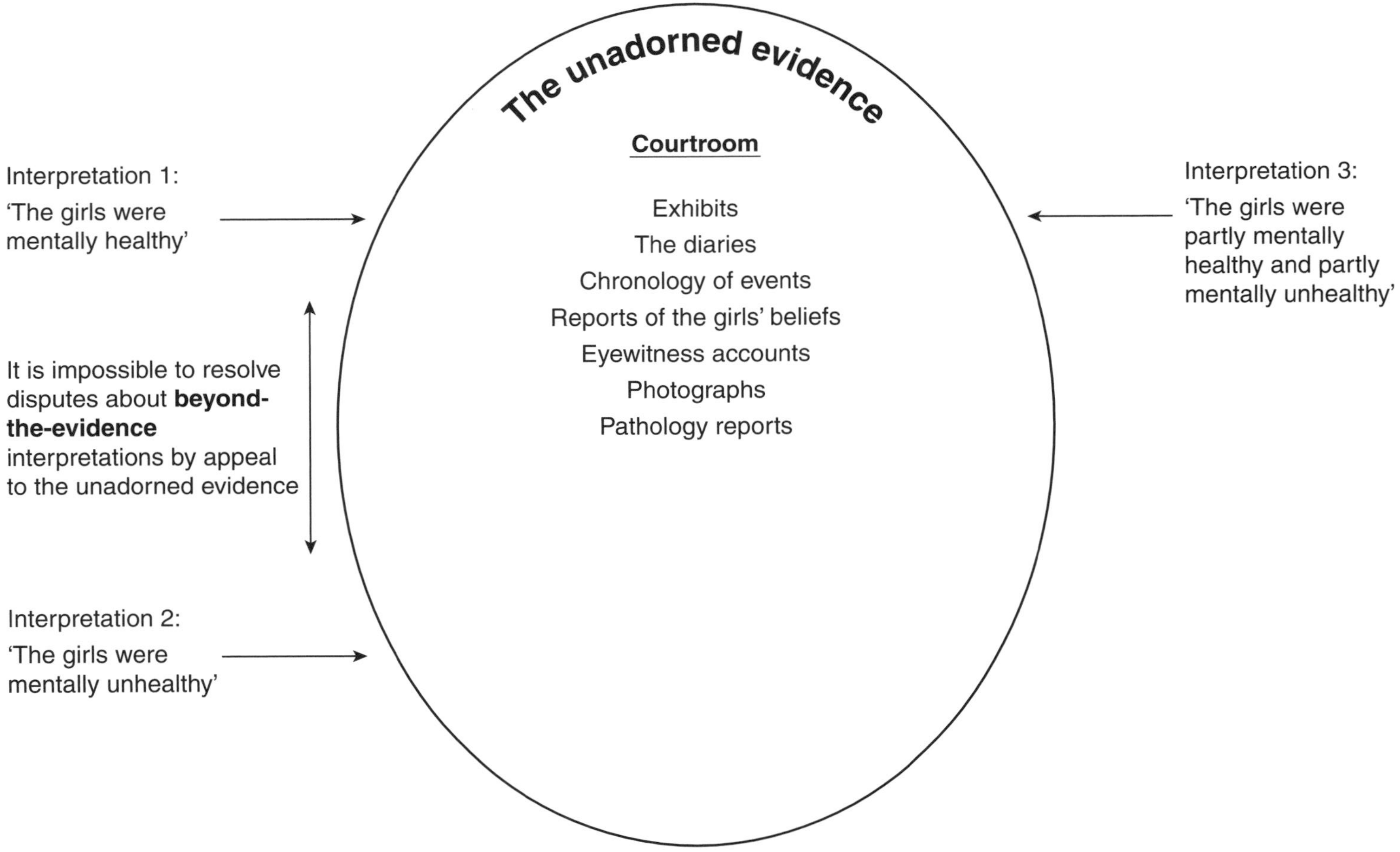
The unadorned evidence
Courtroom
Exhibits
The diaries
Chronology of events
Reports of the girls' beliefs
Eyewitness accounts
Photographs
Pathology reports
Interpretation 1:
'The girls were mentally healthy'
It is impossible to resolve disputes about **beyond-the-evidence** interpretations by appeal to the unadorned evidence
Interpretation 2:
'The girls were mentally unhealthy'
Interpretation 3:
'The girls were partly mentally healthy and partly mentally unhealthy'

Figure 4 Assertions of mental health are always made from beyond-the-evidence

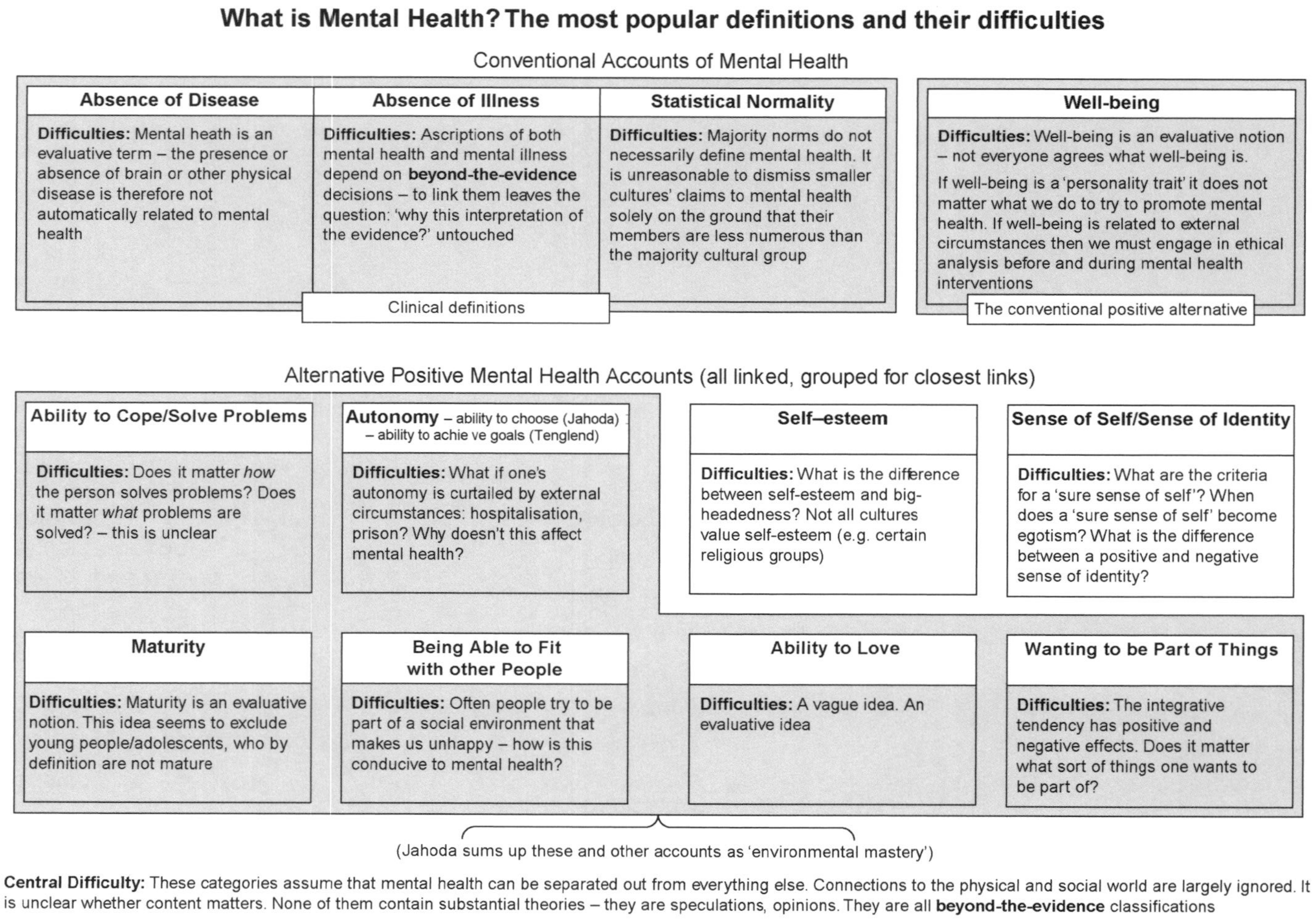
What is Mental Health? The most popular definitions and their difficulties
Conventional Accounts of Mental Health
Absence of Disease
Difficulties: Mental heath is an evaluative term – the presence or absence of brain or other physical disease is therefore not automatically related to mental health
Absence of Illness
Difficulties: Ascriptions of both mental health and mental illness depend on beyond-the-evidence decisions – to link them leaves the question: 'why this interpretation of the evidence?' untouched
Statistical Normality
Difficulties: Majority norms do not necessarily define mental health. It is unreasonable to dismiss smaller cultures' claims to mental health solely on the ground that their members are less numerous than the majority cultural group
Clinical definitions
Well-being
Difficulties: Well-being is an evaluative notion – not everyone agrees what well-being is.
If well-being is a 'personality trait' it does not matter what we do to try to promote mental health. If well-being is related to external circumstances then we must engage in ethical analysis before and during mental health interventions
The conventional positive alternative
Alternative Positive Mental Health Accounts (all linked, grouped for closest links)
Ability to Cope/Solve Problems
Difficulties: Does it matter how the person solves problems? Does it matter what problems are solved? – this is unclear
Autonomy – ability to choose (Jahoda) – ability to achie ve goals (Tenglend)
Difficulties: What if one's autonomy is curtailed by external circumstances: hospitalisation, prison? Why doesn't this affect mental health?
Self–esteem
Difficulties: What is the difference between self-esteem and big-headedness? Not all cultures value self-esteem (e.g. certain religious groups)
Sense of Self/Sense of Identity
Difficulties: What are the criteria for a 'sure sense of self'? When does a 'sure sense of self' become egotism? What is the difference between a positive and negative sense of identity?
Maturity
Difficulties: Maturity is an evaluative notion. This idea seems to exclude young people/adolescents, who by definition are not mature
Being Able to Fit with other People
Difficulties: Often people try to be part of a social environment that makes us unhappy – how is this conducive to mental health?
Ability to Love
Difficulties: A vague idea. An evaluative idea
Wanting to be Part of Things
Difficulties: The integrative tendency has positive and negative effects. Does it matter what sort of things one wants to be part of?
(Jahoda sums up these and other accounts as 'environmental mastery')
Central Difficulty: These categories assume that mental health can be separated out from everything else. Connections to the physical and social world are largely ignored. It is unclear whether content matters. None of them contain substantial theories – they are speculations, opinions. They are all beyond-the-evidence classifications

Figure 5 Conventional and Alternative definitions of Mental Health

disease, statistical normality and well-being. Nevertheless, each has at least one fatal flaw.

WHY MENTAL HEALTH IS NOT THE ABSENCE OF DISEASE

Mental health is not simply the absence of disease because the idea of mental health and the idea of disease are not necessarily related. Disease is typically thought of as a deviation from a statistical norm (though this view is not without its problems[60]) whereas mental health is generally believed to be a positive state that enables people to do well in the social world. Thus, even if a person's brain is abnormal in some way (rendering her *prima facie* mentally diseased/ill) she is not automatically mentally unhealthy because it may still be possible for her to do well in the world – she may, for example, have a brain disease and still possess self-esteem or an ability to cope (both non-disease-based definitions of mental health). Alternatively, society may be organised in such a way that her brain abnormality has a neutral or even positive effect on what she is able to do. For example, it may make her particularly sensitive to the feelings of other people, and this may be highly valued in her society.

Furthermore, while brain disease and injury can obviously affect thoughts and feelings, it is equally true that a host of other factors can do so as well. If you hear that a close friend has become ill you are immediately made unhappy and anxious, quite independently of your brain's pathological status. When you learn she has recovered your consequent happiness is a result of the good news, whether or not you have a brain disease.

WHY IT IS POINTLESS TO DEFINE MENTAL HEALTH AS THE ABSENCE OF MENTAL ILLNESS

Different people, different cultures and different historical periods each define mental illness and mental health in different and sometimes conflicting ways. In the absence of unequivocal **Type 1** evidence (which there can never be in the case of mental health) or a more substantial theory of mental health and illness, there is no progress to be had. The hard questions: Why is this state mental illness? and Why is this state mental health? remain entirely untouched. We are left as we were in the Christchurch courtroom, with different mental health/illness experts disagreeing irreconcilably, because they have nothing more to debate than their different points of view.

WHY MENTAL HEALTH IS NOT STATISTICAL NORMALITY

Statistical normality cannot plausibly define mental health because:

> ...in holding that normality is healthy one either has to take the average of the whole population of the world as normality, or select a smaller group and take their statistical average as a norm.... If we take the whole world population as a starting point we will most likely have to conclude that whole sub-populations are unhealthy...[61]

For example, it is not statistically normal to want to smoke marijuana. However, there are sizeable social groups who regard smoking marijuana as both normal and desirable. To define these people as mentally unhealthy merely because they have a minority habit or desire is both arbitrary and unreasonable.

If you choose a sub-population as definitive of mental health, the problem is worse. If you say, for example, that to be truly mentally healthy you must believe in a Christian God, or Islam, then you condemn everyone else to perpetual lack of mental health – and, of course, you do so beyond any evidence.

WHY WELL-BEING DOES NOT ADEQUATELY DEFINE MENTAL HEALTH

The advocate of well-being as the definition of mental health has three alternatives. She can:

a. keep the notion of mental well-being ambiguous and abstract
b. define it specifically[62]

or

c. permit subjects to define it for themselves.

Each of these options has significant difficulties for practical mental health work. If she keeps the notion vague it is hard to see how the well-being advocate can consistently recommend any practical mental health promotion strategy. If she defines mental well-being specifically then she is plainly making beyond-the-evidence assertions, which not everyone will agree with – immediately creating ethical tensions as she sets out to promote what some people regard as mental health and some others don't. And if the well-being advocate allows subjects to define well-being for themselves some subjects will inevitably specify it in a way the advocate herself will not want to accept.[62]

Marie Jahoda chooses to equate well-being with happiness or satisfaction, but finds difficulties with this idea too:

> First, says Jahoda, there might be external factors that stop people from being happy. War, famine, and environmental hardship are such factors. No one would call somebody mentally ill just because the person is unhappy for reasons like these... [moreover]... what is personally satisfying (interpreted as subjective well-being) is not necessarily socially acceptable, and *vice versa*.[61]

Because of this, Jahoda considers mental health to be a 'personality trait' or 'core personal disposition' separate from a person's physical and social environment. She also takes the view that mental health cannot be a transient phenomenon:

> ...being happy or feeling well for a short period seems to be compatible with mental illness, and being unhappy for a short period is also compatible with positive mental health... many writers instead claim that happiness must be an enduring personality trait in order to be a criterion of health. And Jahoda in the end accepts that happiness or well-being can be seen as a sign of health, but only if it is part of a more or less enduring personality predisposition.[61]

But Jahoda's proposition – that mental health is an enduring disposition to be happy – is not sufficient either. Jahoda believes it inappropriate to call someone mentally ill because external circumstances are making her unhappy (note, in passing, that Jahoda's assumption that mental illness is the opposite of mental health is most confusing since she rejects it elsewhere). But if mental health is not affected by external circumstances then mental health becomes an entirely abstract idea, and therefore practically useless. If we have enduring personality traits to be mentally healthy or not, there is nothing we can do about it (apart from medication, surgery or non-prescription drugs). Furthermore, since Jahoda separates mental health from everything else, the implication is that what actually makes us mentally healthy/happy does not matter. But the cause of a person's happiness or well-being is surely a central ethical and practical issue when it comes to deciding a person's mental health status and intervening to improve it: if a woman is experiencing panic attacks as the result of an abusive relationship then her mental health status is plainly *not* separate from her general life experience, and if health workers are going to do anything to improve her life they must acknowledge that her mental health is not a separate and abstract concept.

THE HEAVENLY CREATURES TEST

In order to think concretely about definitions of mental health we can apply a further test, the **Heavenly Creatures Test**. This is another very simple procedure: if it is possible to say unequivocally that the Heavenly Creatures were mentally healthy or unhealthy according to a particular definition, then we have a solid definition of mental health. If not, we don't.

WERE THE HEAVENLY CREATURES DISEASED AND THEREFORE MENTALLY UNHEALTHY?

No one knows. They may have been. They may have had – they may still have – gross or subtle brain abnormalities that psychiatrists would define as disease. But we cannot be sure, therefore we cannot use this definition to decide whether they were mentally healthy or not.

Test Failed: Inconclusive

WERE THE HEAVENLY CREATURES STATISTICALLY NORMAL AND THEREFORE MENTALLY HEALTHY?

In some senses they were not statistically normal. They had unusually active imaginations and – of course – they murdered someone. But are these abnormalities relevant to a decision about their mental health status? People are complex. We each have an incalculable number of characteristics that might be assessed for statistical normality: height, birth date, religious beliefs, intensity of relationships, ability to focus on goals, type of goal chosen, level of intelligence, coherence of thought, level of recognition of reality... the list is endless. Which of these factors should count in an assessment of mental health?

Moreover, in most senses the girls seem to have been entirely typical of girls their age, only in a few respects were they unusual. Does that make them mentally healthy or unhealthy?

Test Failed: Inconclusive

DID THE HEAVENLY CREATURES HAVE EMOTIONAL WELL-BEING?

Yes and no – it depends what you mean by emotional well-being. Sometimes they were sad, sometimes they were happy, sometimes they were desperate, sometimes they were ecstatic – isn't this what it is like to be a teenager? And when should the assessment of their well-being have been carried out? On the day of the murder? A week before? Six months before? And how would you calculate – during whatever time period you chose – how much and how little well-being they had overall? There are many 'well-being scales' in the literature[63] but they are not identical and they each emanate from beyond-the-evidence (naturally enough, their authors want to make a name for themselves, and so they each come up with different versions).

Certainly, it would be possible to say in crude terms that the Heavenly Creatures didn't have well-being – and to point to what they did as evidence. And yet it would be equally possible to say crudely that they did – how many of us have ever had such a deeply meaningful relationship as they did? What's more – from their point of view – at least until the plan went wrong – *they* defined themselves as having well-being. After all, they were such Heavenly Creatures.

Test Failed: Inconclusive

ALTERNATIVE ACCOUNTS OF MENTAL HEALTH

SENSE OF SELF

There are several alternatives to the absence of disease, statistical normality and well-being ideas. They are briefly described and tested below (they are mostly drawn from Per-Anders Tenglend's book *Mental Health: A Philosophical Analysis*).[61]

Redlich and Freedman[64] claim that the rational adult has three key features: 'a sure sense of the self, of what is psychologically me and not me', 'insight or self-knowledge, and (ability to use) this insight adaptively' and 'self-love and realistic self-esteem', which they try to distinguish from egotism.

THE HEAVENLY CREATURES TEST

Does this mean that the Heavenly Creatures were mentally healthy? Again, it might or it might not. Your opinion is as good as anyone else's. What do you think?

Test Failed: Inconclusive

MATURITY

Rachel Cox[65] posits a similar idea: that mental health is 'the capacity to behave as a coherent unity over time, in a wide variety of situations'. According to Cox, having this inner cohesion or self-consistency is part of being a mature person.

Apparently:

> Mature persons are 'aware of reality', a reality which they can shape, they 'reach out in trust and warmth to other persons', they are 'at peace with themselves', they 'are attentive towards the needs of others', they 'enjoy productivity', and 'tend to grow steadily toward higher levels of competence'.[61]

However, this typically American view of the world and what matters in it is not shared by all cultures.

THE HEAVENLY CREATURES TEST

On this view, the Heavenly Creatures were partly unhealthy and partly healthy – they certainly didn't trust other persons, and would no doubt be described as immature by most adults. However, from their point of view at least, it was quite reasonable for them not to trust other people, since each adult with influence over them truly was conspiring to separate them. This was the reality and they were very much aware of it. Furthermore, they were at peace with themselves (until the adults messed things up), and they were strong, assertive and attentive towards each other's needs.

Test Failed: Inconclusive

ABILITY TO COPE

The ability to cope is often said to be necessary for positive mental health. According to Tenglend, coping might mean:

> ... 'seeking and utilizing of information under stressful conditions', '[regulating] behavior [so] as to optimize simultaneously both the stability of the self structures and their accommodation to environmental requirements', 'problem-solving efforts made by an individual when the demands he faces have a potential outcome of a high degree of relevance for his welfare', 'fitness or ability to carry on those transactions with the environment which result in its maintaining itself, growing or flourishing'.[61]

THE HEAVENLY CREATURES TEST

The girls coped, but not with practical success, and not according to social norms. But they did work out a plan – they undoubtedly did exhibit 'problem-solving efforts ... when the demands [they faced had] a potential outcome of a high degree of relevance for [their] welfare'. Certainly they were not helpless. Perhaps they were simply too inexperienced to be able to cope adequately in the face of so much stress.

Test Failed: Inconclusive

MARIE JAHODA'S CRITERIA FOR POSITIVE MENTAL HEALTH

Marie Jahoda has developed several criteria she considers necessary and sufficient for mental health. In addition to 'well-being as a disposition to be happy' they include:

The ability to be realistically self-reflective

Jahoda believes that the healthy individual should have an 'intact sense of self-hood' and ... be able to look upon herself with detachment. She should be able to compare herself with others objectively and her opinion of herself should be similar to the opinion held of her by others. Essentially, the mentally healthy person should be realistic about herself.

(**Related ideas:** 'maturity', 'sense of self'.)

Balanced feelings about one's own self

Drawing on Maslow's ideas,[66] Jahoda believes healthy persons 'accept themselves and their own nature without chagrin or complaint'. Conversely, it is not healthy to feel bad or inferior for not being perfect: '[a] healthy person knows who he is and does not feel basic doubts about his inner identity'.[67]

(**Related ideas:** 'self-esteem', 'sense of self'.)

Wanting to be part of things

Jahoda also advances the idea of 'investment in living'. This seems to mean being positively concerned with other people, having the capacity to evoke empathic responses from other people, and having long-term significant projects and higher goals in life, plus the motivation to realise them. In other words, the mentally healthy person wants to be part of things.

Autonomy

Autonomy, self-determination, and independence are commonly suggested as criteria of positive mental health. The idea is that the healthy individual is able to make independent decisions, to make 'a conscious discrimination... of environmental factors he wishes to accept or reject'.[68]

In other words, the healthy person is able to take some degree of charge over his environment.

(Note that this is a limited of idea of autonomy. It is only a part of the idea contained in the foundations theory of health described in **Chapter Six**.)

Environmental mastery

Reinforcing the (limited) autonomy idea, Jahoda lists six categories necessary for environmental mastery:

> 1) The ability to love; 2) adequacy in love, work, and play; 3) adequacy in interpersonal relations; 4) efficiency in meeting situational requirements; 5) capacity for adaptation and adjustment; 6) efficiency in problem-solving.[61]

THE HEAVENLY CREATURES TEST

With so many related ideas, and so many nuances, the Heavenly Creatures Test inevitably fits with some, but not all, aspects of Jahoda's thinking.

Test Failed: Inconclusive

TENGLEND'S CRITERIA FOR MENTAL HEALTH

Tenglend's ideas are at least as wide-ranging as Jahoda's. According to Tenglend:

> (A mentally healthy) person has to:
>
> have a high degree of (correct) memory in various senses
> have a high degree of correct perception in both senses
> have a high degree of rationality in three senses
> have a (relatively) high degree of self-knowledge

have some flexibility in two senses
have some ability to experience feelings in general
have some ability to feel empathy in the narrow sense
have some self-esteem and self-confidence
have some ability to communicate cognitive information
have some ability to co-operate[61]

He summarises his list:

> I have argued that the capacity for practical rationality and the ability to co-operate together cover what we mean by acceptable mental health. Together they are sufficient for having the ability to reach basic vital goals, and they are complex enough to encompass all the other abilities discussed and found necessary to some degree. More formally put: P has acceptable mental health iff P has a high degree of practical rationality and some degree of the ability to co-operate.[61]

THE HEAVENLY CREATURES TEST

Tenglend's characterisation seems to pass the Heavenly Creatures Test – the girls were practically rational and they co-operated. Indeed, according to Tenglend's outlook, they appear mentally healthy in virtually every respect (although presumably Tenglend would not agree that killing your mother is a 'vital goal'). However, Tenglend's definition looks plausible only because it is so general – almost all adults, including many of those the psychiatric system defines as mentally ill, are mentally healthy on this account (indeed, so many people are included as mentally healthy it is hard to see what practical difference it makes).

THE FUNDAMENTAL PROBLEM WITH TRYING TO DEFINE MENTAL HEALTH – ALL THE SPECULATIONS FAIL BECAUSE THEY ARE ABSTRACTIONS

We seem to experience mental events as phenomena separate from the physical world. It feels to us that we are self-aware pilots sitting alone in cockpits somewhere inside our individual heads. But even though this is how mental events appear to us, they may not be truly like this. On closer inspection most things turn out to be not what they seem – colour, movement, space, time, the orbiting planets, memory, sentience, altruism, science, intelligence, personality.[69–80] The list is endless, why should 'mind' be just what it seems?

The fundamental problem with trying to define mental health and illness is that it merely reinforces the way the mental appears to us. Any attempt to define mental health must be a process of classifying and valuing (it must be based on **Type 5** and **6** judgements), and if the definer simply accepts the way things seem (that the mental world is disconnected) she is automatically obliged to disconnect the mental from everything else. But this leaves us stuck in a cul-de-sac. It may or may not be true that the mental is separate from the physical, but we will certainly not find out while bound by the view that the mental world is detached. Furthermore, by accepting that the mental is separate from everything else the definer is left with *contentless* notions – she is left with ideas like 'motivation', 'maturity', 'sense of self' and the other categories contained in **Figure 5**, which she can think of only as existing independently – in splendid isolation, concealed within the psychological depths of unique individuals. And yet just a little open-minded reflection shows that these notions do not have a purely independent existence. People are motivated to achieve goals in the physical and social world. We gain maturity not only through abstract reflection – we get it through living the human experience. We discover a sense of self not just by looking inwards to see who we really are, but by listening to what others say about us, observing how they behave towards us, and noticing the ways in which they develop a sense of themselves.

When you think about it just a little more freely, it is obvious that our thoughts are not pure entities, rather they depend on other things and other systems. It might even be argued that they are *nothing more* than the effects of these other systems on the brain.

THE SEDUCTIVE NATURE OF THE BELIEF THAT THE MENTAL IS A SEPARATE REALM

An editor once persuaded me to write a definition of mental health.[81] I came up with this:

> Mental health is a part of the foundations which make up a person's health in general. Sometimes it may make sense to focus solely on a person's mental life, but usually it does not since we are at once physical, mental and social beings.
>
> According to the **foundations understanding of health**:
>
>> Health in general is created by removing obstacles and providing basic conditions in order to help individuals and groups achieve desirable and realistic chosen and biological potentials. **Mental health promotion is** a multi-disciplinary endeavour which works with people and on their environments to foster the achievement or maintenance of the mental strengths people need to deal successfully with life's problems. The prevention and cure of mental disorder may be part of mental health promotion, but is not necessarily a priority.
>
> On this view mental health can be promoted by a theory of health that regards work for health as the thoughtful removal of obstacles in the way of fulfilling biological and chosen human potentials, and by doing anything that can reinforce the foundations. This may include medical therapy, though sometimes medical therapy should be shunned by the health promoter, especially if it appears that it may damage existing foundations.[81]

I tried not to separate mental health promotion from health promotion in general, but I was seduced – I made mental health *part of* the foundations that make up a person's health. But this is an artificial distinction – it is an unexamined **Type 5** classification made from beyond-the-evidence.

Of course it can make sense to set out to promote mental health as if our mental lives are separate from our physical lives. For example, to work to teach a person 'thinking strategies' to cope with feeling depressed, or indeed to work on any of the ideas summarised in the boxes in the lower half of **Figure 5**. However, to act as if there is a separate category called 'the mental' is to shut it and your activities off from all those apparently non-mental things that must contribute to our thoughts, feelings and behaviours. By focusing on abstract ideas, current definitions of mental health ignore or underplay the context in which we must all experience this so-called mental health.

As a result, and because psychiatry activity is so generally associated with mental health, these definitions remain ignored by real world systems – and not least by most current 'mental health services'. If you do not have a realistic, applicable notion of health, health work inevitably becomes dominated by notions of illness and pathology. If you offer practically useless definitions to people trained in therapeutic techniques what else can they do but respond: 'If you can't tell me how to promote health holistically at least I can promote it in my specific way, by working against disease and illness'?

For these and other reasons explained in the remainder of this book, abstract definitions of mental health should be avoided like the plague.

PART TWO

Rational Fields

(and how to use them to promote health)

CHAPTER FOUR

Mind, Body and the Human Experience

> The first rule of ecology is that everything is connected to everything else.
>
> (Attributed to Barry Commoner)

> . . . of course it is perfectly legitimate, and in fact indispensable, for the scientist to try to analyse complex phenomena into their constituent elements – provided he remains conscious of the fact that in the course of analysis something essential is always lost, and its attributes as a whole are more complex than the attributes of the parts.
>
> (Arthur Koestler (1979) *Janus: A Summing Up*, Pan Books)

SUMMARY

This chapter:

- Builds on **Part One**, which described some of the ways in which we file reality, and showed how easy it is for us to assume that our particular filing systems are the final word
- Explains why we should think of the world as fundamentally interconnected, rather than made up of preordained packages
- Gives reasons why we should not automatically separate the mental from the physical
- Argues for open-mindedness, so laying the groundwork for the discussion of rational fields

◆

Part One of *Total Health Promotion* began with an investigation into what can happen when something seemingly goes wrong with the mental life. **Part Two** begins with a brief account of what can happen when something goes wrong with our brains.

The Hip Bone's Connected to the Thigh Bone . . . the Thigh Bone's Connected to the Body . . . the Body's Connected to the Mind . . . the Mind's Connected to the Physical World . . . the Physical World's Connected to the Social World . . .

The popular book on neuroscience – *Descartes' Error* by Antonio Damasio[82] – begins with the strange and rather compelling case of Phineas Gage.

According to Damasio, Phineas Gage was a 'most efficient and capable man', a construction foreman in charge of blasting stone away to construct a new railroad in Vermont in 1848. Gage suffered an accident in which a tamping iron (3 feet 7 inches long, one and a quarter inches in diameter, tapering to one quarter inch) was blown through his left cheek, traversed the front of his brain, and exited at high speed through the top of his head (covered in blood and brains) to land more than 100 feet away.

Amazingly, Gage recovered. He regained his physical strength. He could touch, hear, and see. He walked firmly, used his hands with dexterity and had no noticeable difficulty with speech or language. He could calculate just as well as ever. And yet, as his doctor recounted, the: '...equilibrium or balance, so to speak, between his intellectual faculty and animal propensities'[82] had been destroyed. He was now:

> ...fitful, irreverent, indulging at times in the grossest profanity which was not previously his custom, manifesting but little deference for his fellows, impatient of restraint or advice when it conflicts with his desires, at times pertinaciously obstinate, yet capricious and vacillating, devising many plans of future operation, which are no sooner arranged than they are abandoned...[82]

Damasio explains that:

> While other cases of neurological damage that occurred at about the same time revealed that the brain was the foundation for language, perception and motor function...Gage's story hinted [that]...somehow there were systems in the human brain dedicated more to reasoning than to anything else, and in particular to the personal and social dimensions of reasoning. The observance of previously acquired social convention and ethical rules could be lost as a result of brain damage, even when neither basic intellect nor language seemed compromised. ...[T]he alterations in Gage's personality were not subtle. He could not make good choices, and the choices he made were not simply neutral...one might venture that either his value system was now different, or, if it was still the same, there was no way in which the old values could influence his decisions...Gage lost something uniquely human, the ability to plan his future as a social being.[82]

In short, Gage's intellectual reasoning was as able as ever – he was entirely rational in a logical sense – but he was emotionally and socially incompetent. He could no longer match his logical reasoning to his social contexts and so went from riches to rags, to die a few years after his accident, friendless and in poverty.

Taking his lead from the Phineas Gage case, Damasio describes accumulating evidence that we should recognise what he calls 'the limits of pure reason' – that the intellect alone is not sufficient for us to get on in the social world. Drawing on increasing speculation in contemporary neuroscience, Damasio posits that we are not conscious minds in unconscious bodies (the view he dubs 'Descartes' Error'). Rather we think *somatically* – our bodily responses are *part of* our mental reactions to events. The parts of the brain necessary for balanced reasoning are the parts that connect our bodily responses to our emotional ones.

Damasio's tentative theory is that Gage-like brain damage (he has researched other patients with tumours or damage to the same part of the brain) seems to prevent people properly processing the somatic components of reason. He says:

> Imagine meeting a friend whom you have not seen for a long time...what happens to you, neurobiologically, as that emotion occurs? What does it really mean to 'experience an emotion'?...there is a change in your body state defined by several modifications in different body regions...your heart may race, your skin may flush, the muscles in your

> face change around the mouth and eyes to design a happy expression... there are changes in a number of parameters in the function of viscera (heart, lungs, gut, skin)...[83]

He argues that the:

> ...emotional processing impaired in patients with prefrontal damage...[means that] these patients cannot generate emotions relative to the images conjured up by certain categories of situation and stimuli...[83]

In other words, the link between the bodily experiences and the formation of appropriate emotions has been broken.

Damasio considers that:

> The action of biological drives, body states, and emotions may be an indispensable foundation for rationality. The lower levels in the neural edifice of reason are the same that regulate the processing of emotions and feelings, along with global functions of the body proper such that the organism can survive...Rationality is probably shaped and modulated by body signals, even as it performs the most sublime distinctions and acts accordingly.[84]

This leads him to what he calls the 'somatic-marker hypothesis', which we unconsciously experience as we make choices about how to act:

> '...the key components (of the choice in question) unfold in our minds instantly, sketchily, and virtually simultaneously, too fast for the details to be clearly defined. But now, imagine that *before* you apply any kind of cost/benefit analysis to the premises, and before you reason toward the solution of the problem, something quite important happens: when the bad outcome connected with a given response option comes into mind, however fleetingly, you experience an unpleasant gut feeling [Damasio calls this a somatic marker]...
>
> What does the *somatic marker* achieve? It forces attention on the negative outcome to which a given action may lead, and functions as an automated alarm signal: Beware of danger ahead if you choose the option which leads to this outcome. The signal may lead you to reject, *immediately*, the negative course of action...allow[ing] you *to choose from among fewer alternatives*. There is still room for using a cost/benefit analysis and proper deductive competence, but only *after* the automated step drastically reduces the number of options.[85]

Damasio – and many of his peers in neuroscience – are drawing attention to the fact that although it may seem to us that we are only doing one particular thing at one particular time – kicking a ball, typing a word, thinking about what to say – we are actually doing very many connected things. As I kick a ball in a soccer game I may be anxious or excited, I may have images of my team-mates in mind, and I will remember the last time I tried a similar move. As I type a word I am acting physically, but I may also be exhausted or ecstatic – I may be copy-typing or I may momentarily believe that I am writing something original and interesting. As I think about what to say I may be sweating, I may be remembering, I may be pulling at my hair, I may be thinking of cheating in some way, and I will be aware that what I eventually submit will be seen by others, so I will be deliberately cautious, or reckless or whatever I want to appear. I will know that I am being watched and will act accordingly.

Damasio's commonplace examples of what it is like to experience an emotion reintroduce us to the obvious – they remind us that as our bodies react to danger, for example, we experience physical, emotional and conscious change all at once. Indeed, if you think of any everyday human experience, even the classifications 'physical', 'emotional' and 'conscious' are insecure. We have separate words and ideas for these categories (we even have separate disciplines that research and teach them) but are they *really* separate? I think there is room for doubt.

The more exciting incidents illustrate the point best (though any human experience will do). For example, imagine attending a crowded soccer game where it matters intensely to you and everyone else around you that your team wins in order to secure promotion. It's 0–0 and there are five minutes to go. You and everyone else have steadily become more and more despondent as the game has worn on. It looks like the boys won't score if they play until Wednesday week. Then your team flukes a corner. There's a goalmouth scramble. The ball bounces tantalisingly out to your unmarked centre-forward. His shot rockets the ball into the top corner of the net. You spontaneously hug the stranger next to you. All you can hear are cheers, and all you can feel is heat and breath and jostling – at that moment you do not think of yourself as separate from anything. In fact you do not think of yourself at all – you are there physically *and* emotionally and it would be arbitrary to separate out the emotional bits from the physical ones. Your happiness *is* your experience and your experience *is* your happiness.

This essential interconnectedness (that we habitually deny as we classify reality) can be found in two forms in the Phineas Gage example. There is Damasio's interpretation that Gage's accident destroyed the part of the brain that links the 'somatic marker' to the part of the brain that processes emotions, and therefore disabled Gage's ability to act in a socially connected fashion. And there is the further point that Damasio's 'somatic marker' is not an independent thing either. Whether you have a pleasant or unpleasant experience as the result of a social behaviour depends both on the behaviour *and* its social context. Phineas Gage's changed behaviours were perceived as unwelcome by a social system that didn't value his uncompromising rationality. But another system might conceivably have valued the changed Gage differently. (For example, Phineas might well have made a fine mercenary soldier. Maybe he should have joined the French Foreign Legion.)

REASONS WHY WE SHOULD NOT SEPARATE MINDS FROM BODIES

Damasio's speculations help refocus our interest in the world. We are so used to thinking that Specialist A is expert on Subject A, Specialist B is expert on Subject B and so on, that it can seem to us that the entire world is locked up in sealed boxes, each accessible only to a very few people, and hardly a single one of them accessible to most of us. There is some truth in this, of course. The modern world does require special skills and knowledge that take so long to learn that there is little time to learn anything else properly. However, just because things have become increasingly complex, this does not mean they really are segregated.

Study of the effects of pollution on the environment,[86] and work in chaos theory,[87] for example, shows that actions in one area are rarely if ever restricted to that area alone. And yet we persist with *apparently* obvious and therefore rarely examined distinctions between mental disease and mental illness, mental health and mental illness, psychiatric medicine and non-psychiatric medicine, mind and body, mental health promotion and the rest of health promotion. However, not only is it certain that we can make alternative classifications if we want to, but there are numerous reasons why we should seriously examine our conditioned reflex to separate minds from bodies.

MIND MAY BE A FICTION

There is a huge literature on the philosophy of mind. Philosophers have advanced every conceivable connection and disconnection between mind and body – from the idea that minds and bodies are entirely separate entities[88] to the idea that everything is body.[89] No one knows which of these points of view is actually true – nor does anyone know how to prove one point of view ahead of any other, since each is essentially a **Type 5** classification/speculation.[90] However, it is at least plausible that mind does not really exist, and there are many philosophical arguments to this effect.

CONTEMPORARY NEUROBIOLOGY

As we have seen, work in neurobiology is increasingly indicating that people's mental lives are inseparable from their physical being. This view is supported by research in several other disciplines. For example our understanding of personality, childhood development and gender paints a similar picture.[91–93] The idea, in short, is that the way we are wired-up bodily and what happens to us – how we are raised, how we experience each day, where we live, what race we are, what money we have, how our parents treat us – *both* play an indispensable part in forming our mental lives. Alter the wiring, or take any of the other influences away, and our mental lives change as a consequence.[94]

WHAT IT REALLY MEANS TO EXPERIENCE MENTAL ILLNESS

Jo Ann Walton asked people diagnosed as schizophrenic what being mentally ill feels like. Their replies point relentlessly to the view that schizophrenia is not something experienced in 'little bits', and it is certainly not something that happens only to the mental bit of us:

> Both illness and treatment affect the whole of one's Being. Although schizophrenia is thought of as primarily a mental illness, in fact it has major effects on the body as it is lived, as do hospitalisation, drugs and other therapies such as ECT (electroconvulsive therapy). There is no way to separate, for instance, the sensation of hearing voices from the experience of hearing, nor is there a way to separate visual hallucinations from the experience of sight, or tiredness or fear from an experience of body, mind and spirit together. One hears voices, sees things, feels tired, anxious, restless or afraid. Each of these symptoms is an experience that affects Being-in-the-world as a whole.
>
> Different symptoms bothered participants to varying degrees. No two participants had identical symptoms, although several were described in very similar ways. Since all the participants were taking medication it would be difficult to determine in any objective way which symptoms and experiences were related to illness and which to treatment, and to what degree... having the illness meant that all the participants took regular

medication, so both the illness and its treatment had, at the time of the study, become part of their Being-in-the-world...

Lucy suffered from frightening hallucinations when she was most unwell and, as she explained, she still occasionally experiences some of these sensations. She began by describing how real the voices sounded...

> Because they're so normal sounding, well it's not normal...but because they're so clear and coherent you think well...sometimes you get embarrassed because you think, cor, everybody's listening to that. And why isn't anybody going red, you know, things like that. Sometimes they do it now and it's just a silly little kind of thing. Cos I probably get visions worse than voices now. But it's in a very obscure way like in trees and like I used to, when I used to walk to the dairy or just up the road, I'd have a thing about rats. I'd stand on rats, you know, things like that. And you feel them squish between your toes. So then I'd never walk barefoot for years because I'd think, 'Shit, I'm going to stand on another bloody rat.'...

Jack does not hear voices but there are times when he experiences strange visual images:

> (What happens while you're hallucinating? What sort of things?)
>
> Oh just jagged yellow lines, all queer and then me [sic] brain goes...Part of me brain wants to go to sleep and part of it's frightened to go to sleep. It's horrible and I get horrible bizarre pictures in me brain but I usually get to sleep sooner or later and then sleep it off.[31]

There is the **just is** evidence – the patients' experiences in this case – and then there are **Type 5** choices to classify them one way or another. Conventionally we separate out the mental experiences from the physical ones, but we don't have to. It makes at least as much sense, if not more, to see them as a whole, with changing aspects (in the way that a crowd of people in a sports stadium is a changing whole, with various aspects – singing, cheering, colour, movement – that cannot exist without that particular whole).

What's more, the experiences of the patients are themselves part of and also affected by a yet larger context:

> A group of British researchers conducted a follow-up study of 532 patients discharged from hospital care in Harrow over a 10-year period. Summing up their findings [the authors commented] on the heterogeneous nature of schizophrenia and how this was evident in the lives and characteristics of the people they followed up. While not all the patients had fared badly, unemployment was common, as were social difficulties and restricted lifestyle...
>
> In the month prior to their study, 13.8% of the participants had not done any shopping and 44% had not entered a social setting (such as a café, cinema, or church) where they might make contact with others. Even more disturbing, during the same 1-month period over one fifth of the participants (22%) had had no visitors...For people with schizophrenia, sometimes it is problems arising from the social dimensions of life that lead to rehospitalisation...[95]

Mental illness is a mental, physical, social, spiritual, existential experience – it is about making sense of – and at the very least working out how to survive – a world in which you don't fit, indeed a world that appears to be openly hostile to you. How could it be about anything else? How could being mentally ill not be part of a general human experience, given that it is experienced by complex social beings?

MIND/BODY SCIENCE

The experience of connectedness is all around us, once we free ourselves of our separatist preconceptions. For example, while writing this book I have become unpleasantly aware of the commonplace notion of 'stress' and its effects. I set myself a very demanding deadline to complete the book – a stupid deadline, truth be told – and unsurprisingly began to feel less than ideally well as the deadline loomed ever larger. I began to get tingling hands, I became more irritable than usual, I slept only lightly, I lost energy, my appetite diminished, I couldn't think as clearly as I'm used to, and I got an upset stomach. Wondering what could be wrong with me I hit on a collection of websites about 'stress' – any internet search will reveal many – and I seemed to have every possible symptom.

All these sites talk about the 'physical effects' (like those above) of 'mental' stress. But this is **Type 5** talk. Seen another way – as I have come to see it – it isn't my mind and my body that are stressed – I am stressed, and I am stressed not only because of my writing decision but because of all the other things around me (in particular, two much-loved little children and a busy workload besides my book). If I change any one of the supposedly separate fields – my social life, my mental life or my physical life – this might be seen as 'having an impact on' the other fields. If I were to take a holiday from my other work for example, or if I decide to sleep for two weeks, then of course this would influence the other aspects. However, it makes just as much sense to say that these things are all part of each other – they are all one. Just as if I were to be dismissed from my day job, or I were to win the Lottery, it wouldn't be just a bit of me affected – it would be all of me.

There is a growing literature on 'mind/body links', some of which is listed below. Most of it is taken from http://healthhelper.com/complementary/book_mb/intro.htm[96]

The website opens like this:

> **Meaning of mind-body**
> Any discussion of mind-body interventions brings the old questions back to life: What are mind and consciousness? How and where do they originate? How are they related to the physical body? In approaching the field of mind-body interventions, it is important that the mind not be viewed as if it were dualistically isolated from the body, as if it were doing something to the body. Mind-body relations are always mutual and bidirectional – the body affects the mind and is affected by it. **Mind and body are so integrally related that, in practice, it makes little sense to refer to therapies as solely 'mental' or 'physical'**...
>
> When the term mind-body is used in this report, therefore, there is no implication that an object or thing – the mind – is somehow acting on a separate entity – the body. **Rather, 'mind-body' could perhaps best be regarded as an overall process that is not easily dissected into separate and distinct components or parts.** This point of view, which was put forward a century ago by William James, the father of American psychology, has recently been reaffirmed by brain researchers Francis Crick and Christof Koch (1992).[96]
> (Bold mine)

It makes more sense and it is more in keeping with the raw evidence to talk of the *human experience*, rather than separate minds and bodies.

At the very least, exploring interconnectedness is a potential mine of medical progress:

> Most traditional medical systems appreciate and make use of the extraordinary interconnectedness of the mind and the body and power of each to affect the other. In contrast, modern Western medicine has regarded these connections as of secondary importance...
>
> During the past 30 years, there has been a powerful scientific movement to explore the mind's capacity to affect the body and to rediscover the ways in which it permeates and is affected by all of the body's functions...
>
> During the same time, medical researchers have discovered other cultures' healing systems, such as meditation, yoga, and tai chi, which are grounded in an understanding of the power of mind and body to affect one another; developed techniques such as biofeedback and visual imagery, which are capable of facilitating the mind's capacity to affect the body; and examined some of the specific links between mental processes and autonomic, immune, and nervous system functioning – most dramatically illustrated by the growth of a new discipline, psychoneuroimmunology...
>
> From this perspective it is becoming clear that every interaction between doctors and patients – between those who give help and those who receive it – may affect the mind and in turn the body of the patient.[96]

This ought to be no surprise at all. For example, it **just is** a matter of fact that your blood pressure tends to rise when you go to see the doctor.[97] As it does you rehearse what you are going to say, you get anxious, you fluff your lines, you feel embarrassed, you may be in pain – all these things are not little bits that are really separate – they *are* your experience.

I could explain my experience as a writer of philosophy books for health workers as a purely intellectual matter. After all, philosophers are supposed to think free from distractions, in a logical realm removed from the imperfections of the human experience. But if I did it would be a lie – or at least a hopeless caricature of my real experience. Certainly, I do what I do in part as a logical and intellectual challenge. However, it is also true that the reasons I do it are inextricably related to my experience of parental sickness, the effects of which still, decades later, affect me and my siblings. If I am even a little bit truthful I also write to be respected, to tire myself out, to feel that I've achieved something, to feed and protect my wife and children, to have a career, to feel that I belong, to help other people and to be aggressive toward what I see as stupidity – and stupidity affects me physically (there is a lot of it about, and it makes me very angry). Furthermore, the foundations theory of health – which is briefly summarised in **Chapter Five** – has not developed only as a matter of logic, it has come into being mostly as a result of my growing up in reasonable comfort in a welfare state.[63] My philosophy is not pure – if its only source were in 'pure reason' there would be no philosophy at all.

Indeed, sometimes my philosophy is physically unavoidable. It doesn't happen often, unfortunately, but occasionally I wake up with an idea that I must write down, or I relax in the shower and get some sort of solution to a problem that has been bothering me. If I don't write it down quickly – if the kids interrupt me, for instance – I become snappy, stressed, I imagine my blood pressure rises, certainly my pulse quickens. My philosophy is part of ME as a whole, and I am part of all those things that have formed me and form me still.

In just the same way it is an error – and a pervasive one at that – to separate out 'ethical issues' from 'technical matters' or 'purely clinical judgement'. There is a widespread myth abroad that most of what happens in health care happens in an ethical vacuum – that health care is a technical process in which ethics is irrelevant. According to this ridiculous view, ethics matters only in those dramatic cases where doctors and nurses face hard dilemmas. But this is just another inadequate **Type 5** separation. If you take the alternative view, as I do,[98] that the basic question of ethics is 'how should I act in the presence of other lives?' then every interaction between doctor and patient has ethical content – and the separation of ethics from non-ethics is both damaging and distressingly artificial.

Even medical scientists are at last coming to see these interconnections:

> **Evidence of Mind-Body Effects in Contemporary Medical Science**
> **Social isolation**. Biological scientists have long been aware of the importance of social relationships on health. As the evolutionary biologist George Gaylord Simpson observed, 'No animal or plant lives alone or is self-sustaining. All live in communities including other members of their own species and also a number, usually a large variety, of other sorts of animals and plants. The quest to be alone is indeed a futile one, never successfully followed in the history of life.[99]
>
> This observation is nowhere truer than in the human domain, where perceptions of social isolation and aloneness may set in motion mind-body events of life-or-death importance. This point has been demonstrated in research on many dimensions of human experience, among them the following:
>
> **Bereavement**. The idea that a person can die from being separated suddenly from a loved one is rooted in history and spans all cultures – the 'broken heart' syndrome. In the United States, 700,000 people aged 50 or older lose their spouses annually. Of these, 35,000 die during the first year after the spouse's death. Researcher Steven Schleifer of Mount Sinai Hospital, New York, calculates that 20 percent, or 7000, of these deaths are directly caused by the loss of the spouse. The physiological processes responsible for increased mortality during bereavement have been the subject of extensive investigations and include profound alterations in cardiovascular and immunological responses. In study after study, the mortality of the surviving spouse during the first year of bereavement has been found to be 2 to 12 times that of married people the same age...
>
> **Poor education and illiteracy**. A more general and pervasive form of isolation results from poor education and illiteracy, which are in turn associated with increased incidence of disease and death...
>
> Many believe that the common factor in poor education, poor health, and higher mortality is simply that the poorly educated take worse care of themselves. However, research shows that smoking, exercise, diet, and accessibility to health care, while important, do not explain the poorer health and earlier death of these people; the influence of social isolation and poor education is more powerful...
>
> The underlying pathophysiological processes by which social isolation may bring about poor health have been illuminated by studies of primates in the wild. Low-ranking baboons, whose entire life is spent in constant danger with little control, demonstrate high circulating levels of hydrocortisone, which remain elevated even when the stressful event has passed...
>
> **Work status**. Attitude toward work and work status may also be intimately related to health and well-being. Several lines of evidence point to these correlations:
>
> • Robert A. Karasek and colleagues have shown that the job characteristics of high demand and low decision latitude have predictive value for myocardial infarction. Occupational groups embodying these personality traits – waiters in busy restaurants, assembly line workers, and gas station attendants, for example – are at increased risk for heart attack. Their hypothesis is that increasing job demands are harmful when

environmental constraints prevent optimal coping or when coping does not increase possibilities for personal and professional growth and development...

• Psychologist Suzanne C. Kobasa and colleagues have identified job qualities that offer protection against cardiovascular morbidity and mortality, even in psychologically stressful job settings. They refer to the 'three Cs':

> (1) control – a sense of personal decision-making; (2) challenge – the sense of personal growth and wisdom; becoming a better person; and (3) commitment to life on and off the job – to work, community, family, and self. Persons experiencing these qualities are said to possess 'hardiness' and are relatively immune to job-induced illness or death.[96]

Note that these attributes are reminiscent of the definitions of mental health described in **Chapter Three**. Much more importantly, however, note that they are not independent of other things – having a sense of control depends on actually being able to control things, for example. And being committed to off-the-job life means having the resources to be so committed.

Perceived meaning and health
Perceived meaning – how one perceives an event or issue, what something symbolizes or represents in one's mind – has direct consequences for health...

More recently, careful studies have indicated the pivotal role of perceived meaning in health. Sociologists Ellen Idler of Rutgers University and Stanislav Kasl of the Department of Epidemiology and Public Health at Yale Medical School studied the impact of people's opinions on their health – what their health meant to them. The study involved more than 2800 men and women, and the findings were consistent with the results of five other large studies involving more than 23,000 people. All these studies lead to the same conclusion: One's own opinion about his or her state of health is a better predictor than objective factors, such as physical symptoms, extensive exams, and laboratory tests, or behaviors such as cigarette smoking. For instance, people who smoked were twice as likely to die during the next 12 years as people who did not, whereas those who said their health was 'poor' were seven times more likely to die than those who said their health was 'excellent'...

Placebo response
• The placebo response is almost ubiquitous. Studies show that in virtually any disease, roughly one-third of all symptoms improve when patients are given a placebo treatment without drugs...[96]

CONCLUSION

We have a problem, and we seem to have no way to deal with it:

1. The world and its interrelationships are (probably inconceivably) complex.
2. In order to understand, explain and indeed do anything within this vast complexity we have to select little bits of the world rather than the whole thing (this book, for example, is an argument for a form of holism, but inevitably it must choose only the most meagre selection of examples, points to argue, and words from the dictionary).
3. This inevitable selection process leads to two things:
   a. the belief that the selected aspects actually are separate;
   b. specialisms and tribes of specialists.

4. If the world isn't actually separate then, as we select little bits of it, we surround ourselves with theoretical barriers that are, paradoxically both necessary (for us to understand anything) and unnecessary (since it is we who add them to the evidence).
5. We therefore need to find a way that will allow us to think and practise holistically without having to attempt the impossibility of having to think of everything at once – we need a practical holism that allows us to think of things as separate, while enabling us to remember that it is we who choose to think of them like this.

WE MUST CONSIDER THE HUMAN EXPERIENCE

It should now be clear why it is a mistake to seek to promote mental health separately from health in general, or whatever it is thought to be separate from. The Heavenly Creatures did not simply 'go mad' or 'suffer possession' – or any other of the uni-dimensional explanations we desperately suggest – rather a great range of factors came together to constitute their human experience: their schooling, their relationships, their selfishness, their arrogance, their families, their fantasies, their physical and mental feelings for each other. Being in love is a physical as well as a mental experience – it makes you sick, it makes your heart race – it affects YOU (a big you, all of YOU in capital letters) and it affects other people too – your previous lover, your family, your friends (they laugh at you, they care for you, they are jealous of you). And all this culminated (or at least we say it culminated – their life went on afterwards) in behaviours that were seen as a problem by most people around them.

The point is that we tie ourselves up by thinking of mind and body as separate – this separation is an artefact which we have excessively institutionalised. We must instead consider *the human experience*, and if we want to promote health we must consider how best we can improve this human experience in general.

Once this interconnectedness is acknowledged – and once the ideas of psychiatry, mental illness and mental health – and all the associated verbal paraphernalia – are seen for what they are: as proposals, possible ways amongst countless other possible ways of classifying an interconnected reality – then we are immediately liberated. We can adopt alternative classifications if we wish. And, given the well-documented social and ethical problems created by the conventional classifications, we are surely entitled at least to experiment with alternatives.

Chapter Five explains the background to a practical method for experimenting with alternatives – the idea of rational fields. It explains what rational fields are and how they are formed, it explains that rational fields have different levels of stability, it describes how to detect these different levels of stability, and it shows that psychiatry and conventional mental health promotion are failed or failing rational fields. **Chapter Six** expands the idea. It explains how to create a rational field using a rational field template, shows the value of comparing rational fields with surrounding rational fields, and shows how the creation of rational fields inspired by a theory of health might quickly create a liberating, flexible, autonomy-centred form of health promotion – total health promotion. Rational fields enable us to recognise and act on interconnectedness, permanently 'conscious of the fact that in the course of analysis something essential is always lost'.

CHAPTER FIVE

Rational Fields

SUMMARY

This chapter:

- Explains what rational fields are
- Describes the difference between a natural rational field and a manufactured one
- Shows how a mix of evidence and non-evidence can be combined to create a manufactured rational field
- Explains how to assess the stability of a manufactured rational field
- Presents psychiatry and mental health promotion as examples of manufactured rational fields
- Demonstrates that psychiatry and mental health promotion are both disintegrating rational fields (held together by human instincts, classifications and values)
- Develops the argument that once we are explicit about rational fields and their source in instinct, classification and value, we can be liberated in our health promotion work

INTRODUCTION

Chapter Five explains how our need to think of the world as made up of separate 'little bits' causes us to manufacture rational fields. Rational fields are a problem if we are unaware of their existence. However, once we know what they are and how they are created we are free to make the very most of them. Familiarity with rational fields enables us to recognise the beyond-the-evidence instincts, classifications and values that create and sustain them. We can quickly explain these to other people, and we can also assess and develop rational fields. We can alter them, we can create new ones, we can compare various rational fields, and best of all we can combine elements from different rational fields in order to maximise our health promotion efforts.

This chapter is probably the most difficult in the book. It may be hard to understand, and it is also experimental – the rational field idea will take time to perfect. This is merely an opening attempt to explain it, and its possibilities. Nevertheless, readers are encouraged to grapple with the idea, since an understanding of rational fields is essential to effective total health promotion.

WHAT IS A RATIONAL FIELD?

RATIONAL FIELDS INTRODUCED

All rational fields have the same basic structure.[101–104] They are formed by any kind of problem-solving behaviour, and can therefore be any size from minuscule to enormous. A rational field is initially created either by an instinct or a value-judgement or both. These instincts or judgements generate goals and sub-goals, strategies and sub-strategies, each of which maintains the rational field.

NATURAL AND MANUFACTURED RATIONAL FIELDS

Natural rational fields

It **just is** the case that the living world is composed of innumerable rational fields. A plant is a rational field, striving to grow and to propagate. A bacterium is a rational field, a cell in a body is a rational field, a gene is a rational field, organs in the human body are rational fields, a developing person is a rational field: anything that is instinctively purposive is a natural rational field. All the above examples have goals and sub-goals, strategies and sub-strategies, each of which maintain the rational field. If new problems emerge, each rational field may expand or adapt in order to try to deal with them. For example, in ideal circumstances a plant will grow and produce many seeds. If there is a drought, or if the plant is attacked by insects, or if there is excessive wind, then if it can it will adapt its goals and strategies accordingly (perhaps it will make only one fruit instead of many, or perhaps it will produce special chemicals to repel further insect attack, or perhaps it will grow extra roots as an anchor). The same is true of any natural, goal-directed system.[105]

This **just is** the way the world is – natural rational fields exist within-the-evidence.

A similar observation was made by Arthur Koestler, who believed that:

> A living organism is not an aggregation of elementary parts, and its activities cannot be reduced to elementary 'atoms of behaviour' forming a chain of conditioned responses. In its bodily aspects, the organism is a whole consisting of 'sub-wholes', such as the circulatory system, digestive system, etc., which in turn branch into sub-wholes of a lower order, such as organs and tissues...[100]

Koestler offered the image of a living organism, which he saw as a set of semi-autonomous, interconnected systems, shown in **Figure 6**.

Koestler elaborates:

> ...each member of this hierarchy, on whatever level, is a sub-whole or *'holon'* in its own right – a stable, integrated structure, equipped with self-regulatory devices and enjoying a considerable degree of *autonomy* or self-government. Cells, muscles, nerves, organs, all have their intrinsic rhythms and patterns of activity, often manifested spontaneously

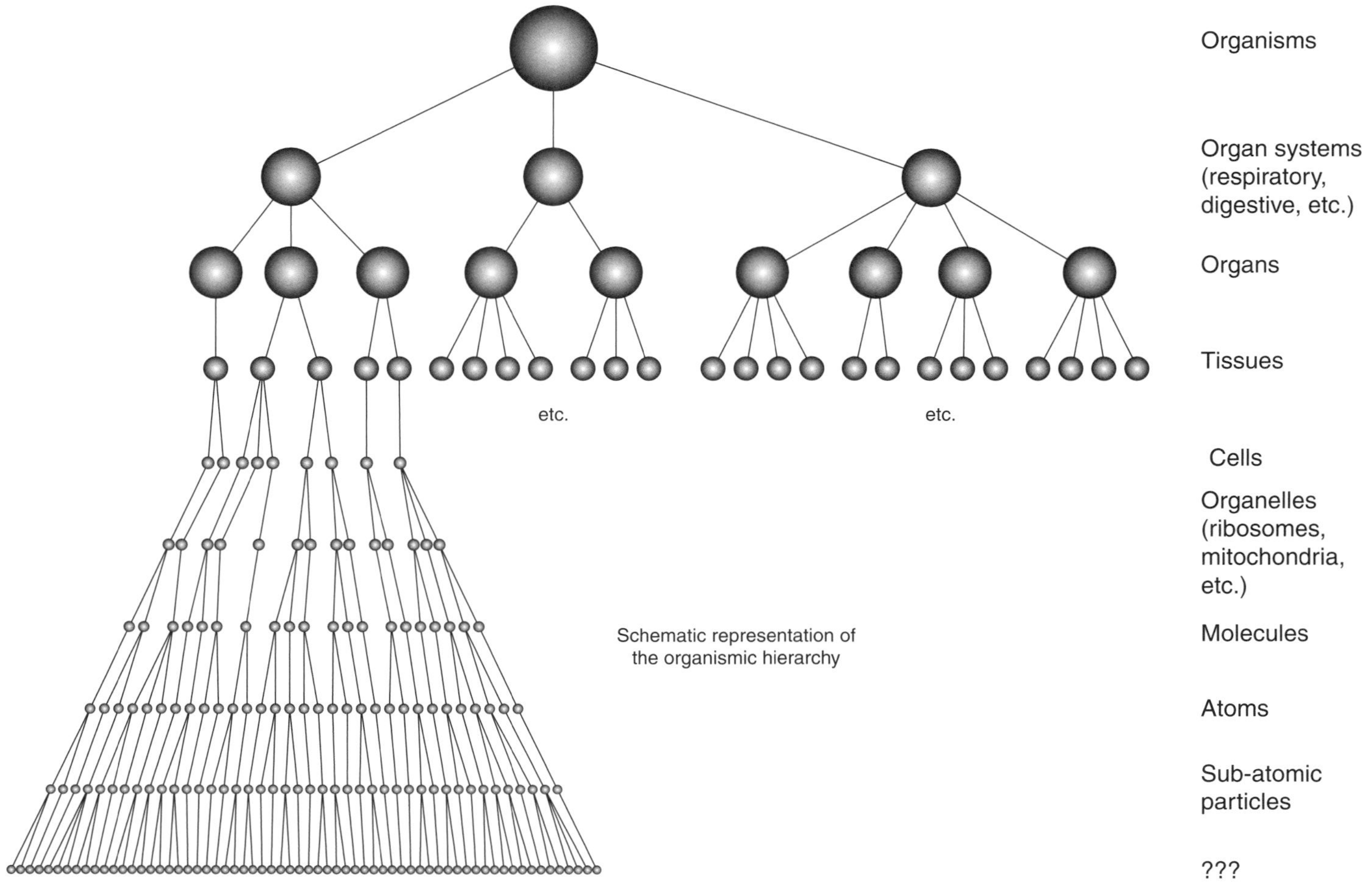

Figure 6 Koestler's 'Schematic representation of the organismic hierarchy'. Reproduced with permission from Koestler, A. (1979). *Janus: A Summing Up*, Pan Books Ltd

> without external stimulation; they are subordinated as *parts* to the higher centres of the hierarchy, but at the same time function as quasi-autonomous *wholes*...[100]

Koestler gave examples of the autonomy of the *holons*: the human heart has several independent pacemakers, a strip of tissue taken from the heart of a chicken embryo and put in nutrient solution will go on pulsating for years, and transplant surgery clearly shows that individual organs can be 'quasi-independent'. Anticipating the developments summarised in **Chapter Four**, Koestler also speculated that:

> Science is only just beginning to rid itself of the mechanistic preconceptions of the nineteenth century – the world as a billiard table of colliding atoms – and to realise that hierarchical organisation is a fundamental principle of living nature...[100]

Natural rational fields are in keeping with Koestler's idea. None are wholly independent – because of the world's interconnectedness – but any rational field must have at least one distinct purpose and a strategy by which to pursue it. Each part of Koestler's *holarchy* exhibits goal-directed activity too, and goal-directed problem-solving activity is the essence of a rational field.

The point of rational fields – and *holons* – is the exercise of autonomy, and the point of other contributing *holons* is to provide the wherewithal for autonomy while being autonomous themselves. Rational fields are not the same as *holons*, at least I don't think they are. A rational field does not have to be seen as part of a hierarchy, and rational fields are often disharmonious, both within themselves and with other rational fields. Nonetheless, rational fields and *holons* obviously have much in common.

Manufactured rational fields

Manufactured rational fields are different from natural ones. They are also goal-directed (they must be to be rational fields), but they tend to be more erratic and unstable than natural rational fields, since they are formed by human beyond-the-evidence assumptions and decisions.

Natural rational fields are all around and even within us, and are rightly of much interest to those health promoters who concentrate on disease prevention and proper biological function. Manufactured rational fields are formed and sustained by *our* classifications of reality (**Type 5**), *our* values (**Type 6**), and *our* instincts (see **Figure 2**). And it is these that are of greatest relevance to total health promotion.

Manufactured rational fields can be as small as a plan to read a book with a glass of wine this evening, and as big as it is possible for any human institution to be. Conventional health services are manufactured rational fields, Microsoft is a manufactured rational field, Microsoft's marketing department is a manufactured rational field, and so is psychiatry, nursing, a badminton club, the law – every system designed by humans to achieve a purpose is a manufactured rational field (the Heavenly Creatures established a rational field as they planned to kill Honora Parker).

Once we can properly recognise manufactured rational fields for what they are we can take control over them. Once we know what we are dealing with we do not have to fall into rational fields that suit other people more than they suit us, and we do not have to follow particular goal-directed paths in the false belief that these paths are all there is.

An Example of a Simple Manufactured Rational Field

A traveller unexpectedly lost in a foreign city, unable to speak or read the native language, must define a goal and devise ways to achieve it if she wants to regain her bearings. She might think: I don't want to be lost (a value judgement or instinct which defines the field's perimeter), if I find the central railway station I will probably find a map (two related goals), if I draw a picture of a train with a question mark and show it around I may get directions to the station (two related strategies), first I need to find some paper (sub-goal)... and so on. By doing these things she creates a small rational field. As she formulates and tries strategies to achieve her goal the field expands. As soon as she is successful, the rational field dissipates.

An Example of a Complex Manufactured Rational Field

Large organisations such as hospitals and commercial companies create and perpetuate vast and complex rational fields. Just like the traveller's field, these larger fields are initially created by classifications and value-judgements or instincts (we must treat disease, we must improve our brand recognition) which generate further goals and sub-goals, strategies and sub-strategies, each of which contributes to the rational field's evolution.

To describe the relationships between the goals, strategies and means of an organisation the size of BP is a virtually impossible task – even the most determinedly extensive depiction of BP's rational field would be an oversimplification. But fortunately the exact details don't matter for present purposes. They can be calculated as necessary for any particular total health promotion project – rather it is the basic *structure* and *formation* of rational fields that needs to be understood. If you know this then you can assess any manufactured rational field for coherence and value, and can knowingly manufacture a rational field according to your own classifications and values.

THE RATIONAL FIELD TEMPLATE

All rational fields, whether natural or manufactured, can be very crudely depicted, as in **Figure 7**.

A plant's instinctive rational field response to an attack by an insect might be illustrated as in **Figure 8**.

Figure 8 is a **natural** rational field. Its means are well related to its goals, and its goals are compatible. Some loss of optimal normal functioning is tolerated in order to achieve **Goal Z**.

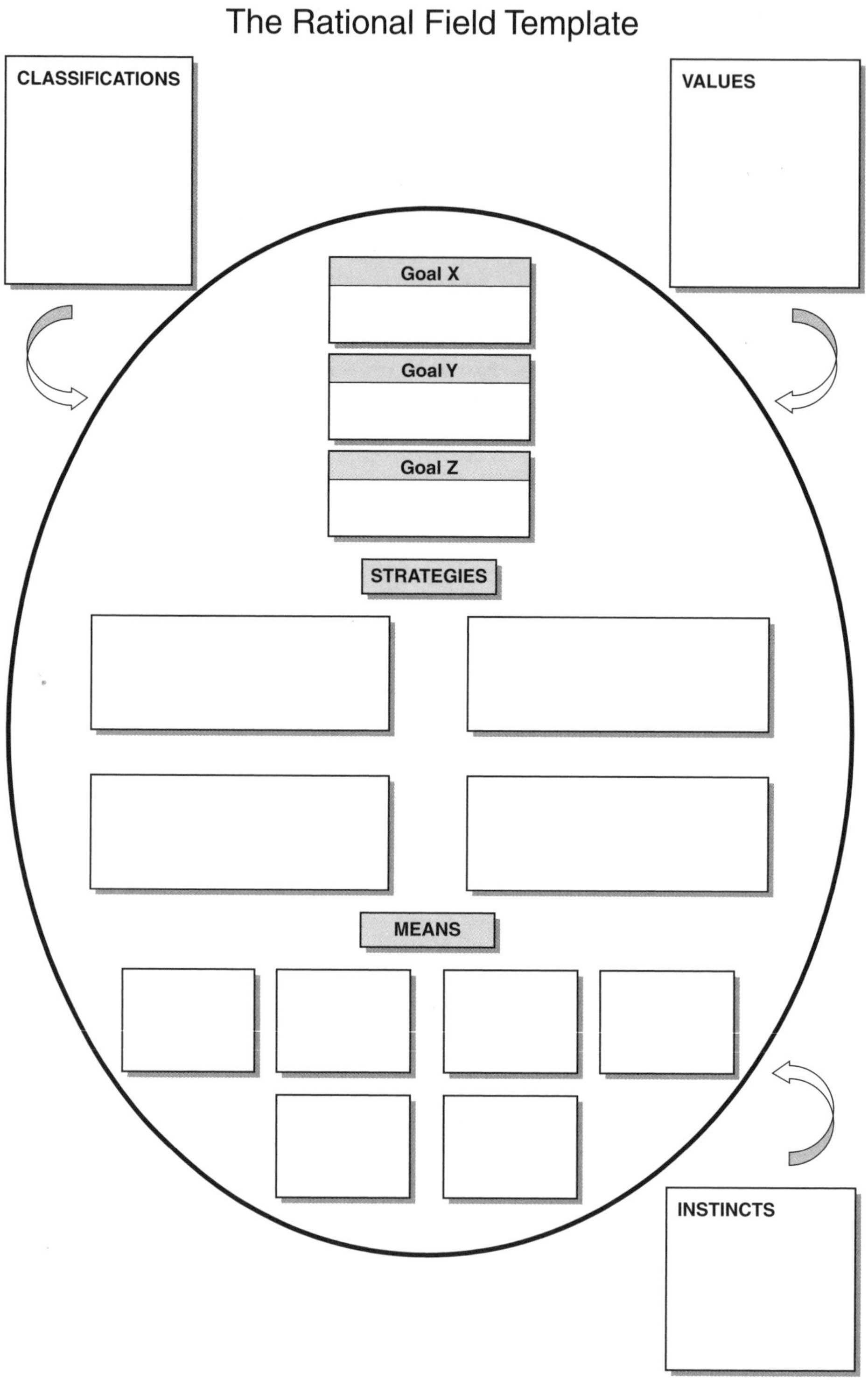

Figure 7 The Basic Rational Field Template

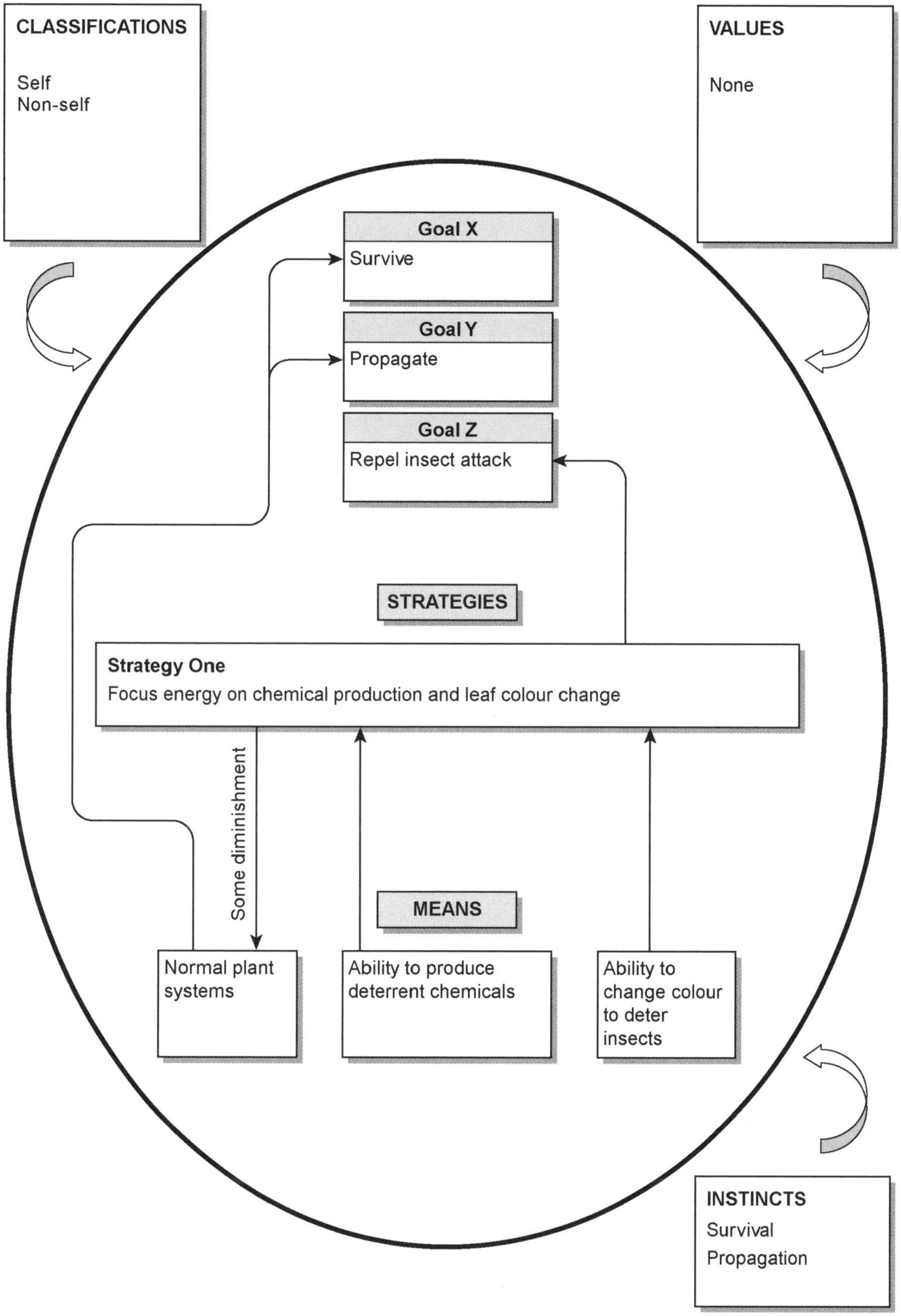

Figure 8 The Rational Field Template simply expressed for a plant's reponse to insect attack (this is a natural rational field)

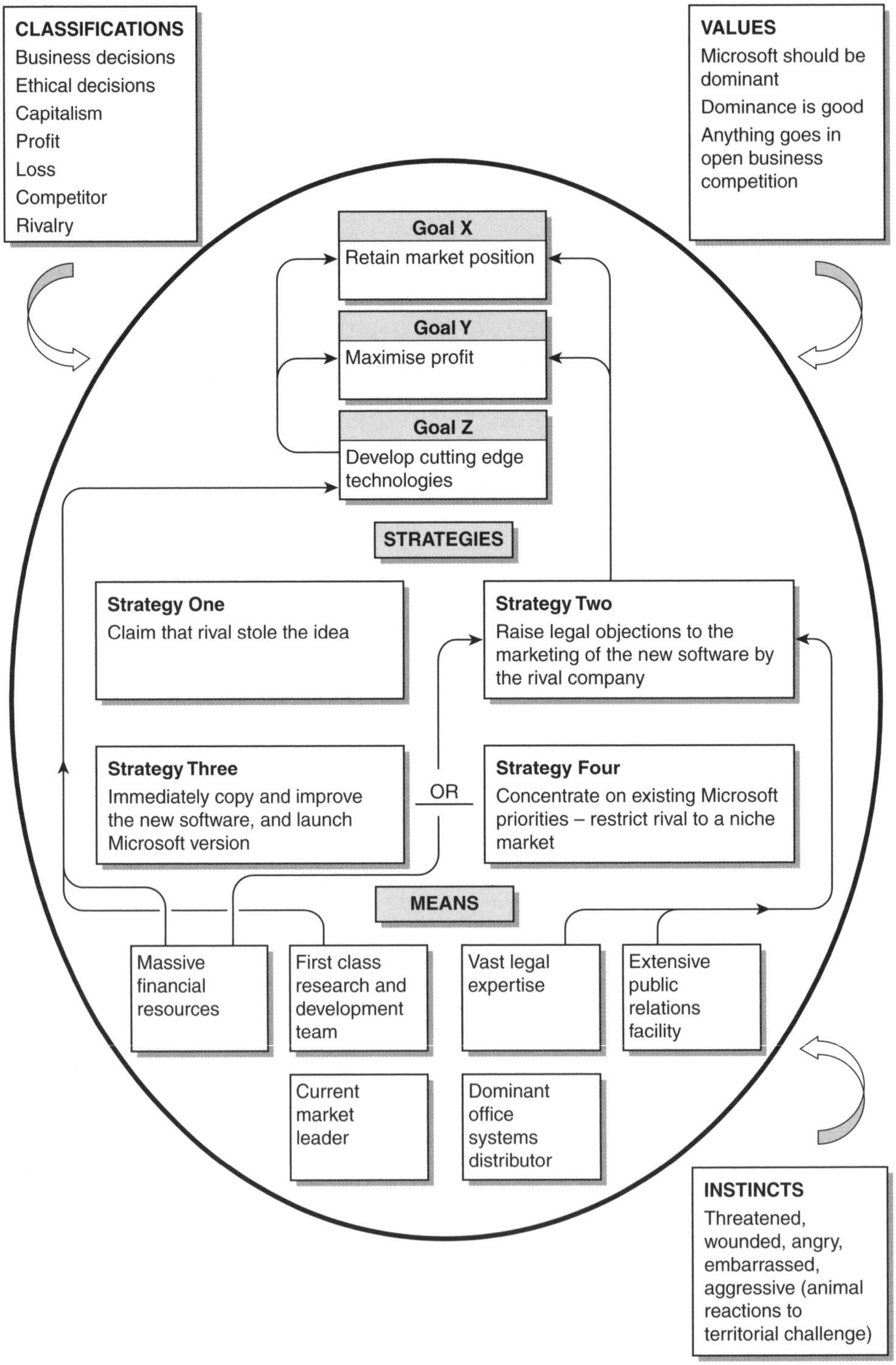
CLASSIFICATIONS
Business decisions
Ethical decisions
Capitalism
Profit
Loss
Competitor
Rivalry
VALUES
Microsoft should be dominant
Dominance is good
Anything goes in open business competition
Goal X
Retain market position
Goal Y
Maximise profit
Goal Z
Develop cutting edge technologies
STRATEGIES
Strategy One
Claim that rival stole the idea
Strategy Two
Raise legal objections to the marketing of the new software by the rival company
Strategy Three
Immediately copy and improve the new software, and launch Microsoft version
OR
Strategy Four
Concentrate on existing Microsoft priorities – restrict rival to a niche market
MEANS
Massive financial resources
First class research and development team
Vast legal expertise
Extensive public relations facility
Current market leader
Dominant office systems distributor
INSTINCTS
Threatened, wounded, angry, embarrassed, aggressive (animal reactions to territorial challenge)

Figure 9 The Rational Field Template crudely expressed for Microsoft's response to a rival company's revolutionary software (this is a manufactured rational field)

Microsoft's **manufactured** rational field response to the surprise emergence of revolutionary software from a rival company might (again very crudely) be illustrated as in **Figure 9**.

In **Figure 9** the company's decision is to adopt Strategy Two, to try to prevent the rival launching its product, in order to give Microsoft time to increase its own research and development efforts. It is not suggested that the solution offered in **Figure 9** is what Microsoft would actually do. Rather, it is an illustrative response, meant only to introduce the idea of a manufactured rational field.

At this stage, the main points to note about rational fields are:

1. That even so simply expressed, the rational field template is useful because it enables decision-makers to state their most important goals, to crudely check whether these goals are compatible with each other, to define and lay out different strategies, to see how these impact on the goals (some may fit with one goal but not another, for example), to state the primary means for achieving any goals, and to assess whether the means, strategies and goals are coherent and efficient.

2. Even more important, it is possible, by using the rational field template, to see how a rational field is formed from beyond-the-evidence. In addition to a simple internal field made up of means, strategies and goals, the rational field template shows three boxes – one for *instincts*, one for *classifications* and one for *values* that help explain why the internal goals and strategies have been selected. Instincts, classifications and values shape the rational field – they form its walls. Usually, in our social affairs, we tend not to notice or we play down these elements. But they are crucial for the rational field template. Only by properly understanding them can we understand our rational fields, and judge between them comprehensively.

Filling in the instinct, value and classification boxes can be an uncomfortable process, particularly for people who have never conceived that their world is an option rather than a necessary reality. To have these very basic human judgements forced into the open can feel like a home invasion (which it is, in a way). But it is necessary if we are to be able to explore our thinking and our policies open-mindedly.

Considerable personal judgement is required to complete the rational field template, and it may therefore be that some people fill in the values, classification and instincts boxes only sparsely, if at all. However, this is a form of denial, and must be overcome for total health promotion to succeed. There very obviously must be values, instincts and choices in play, or else there can be no manufactured rational fields. Users of the rational field template might as well get used to the idea of being honest about their biases. And if this is too much to bear then it can help to get other people – preferably people with different values and a different way of seeing the world – to help fill in the template. This way at least you can begin to decide whether you have been as fully open as you might have been in listing the formative elements of your rational field.

It is also worth noting that there are overlaps between classifications, values and instincts. For example, an instinct is often the basis for a value and valuing things is itself a form of classification (interestingly, the denial of instinct is also a common

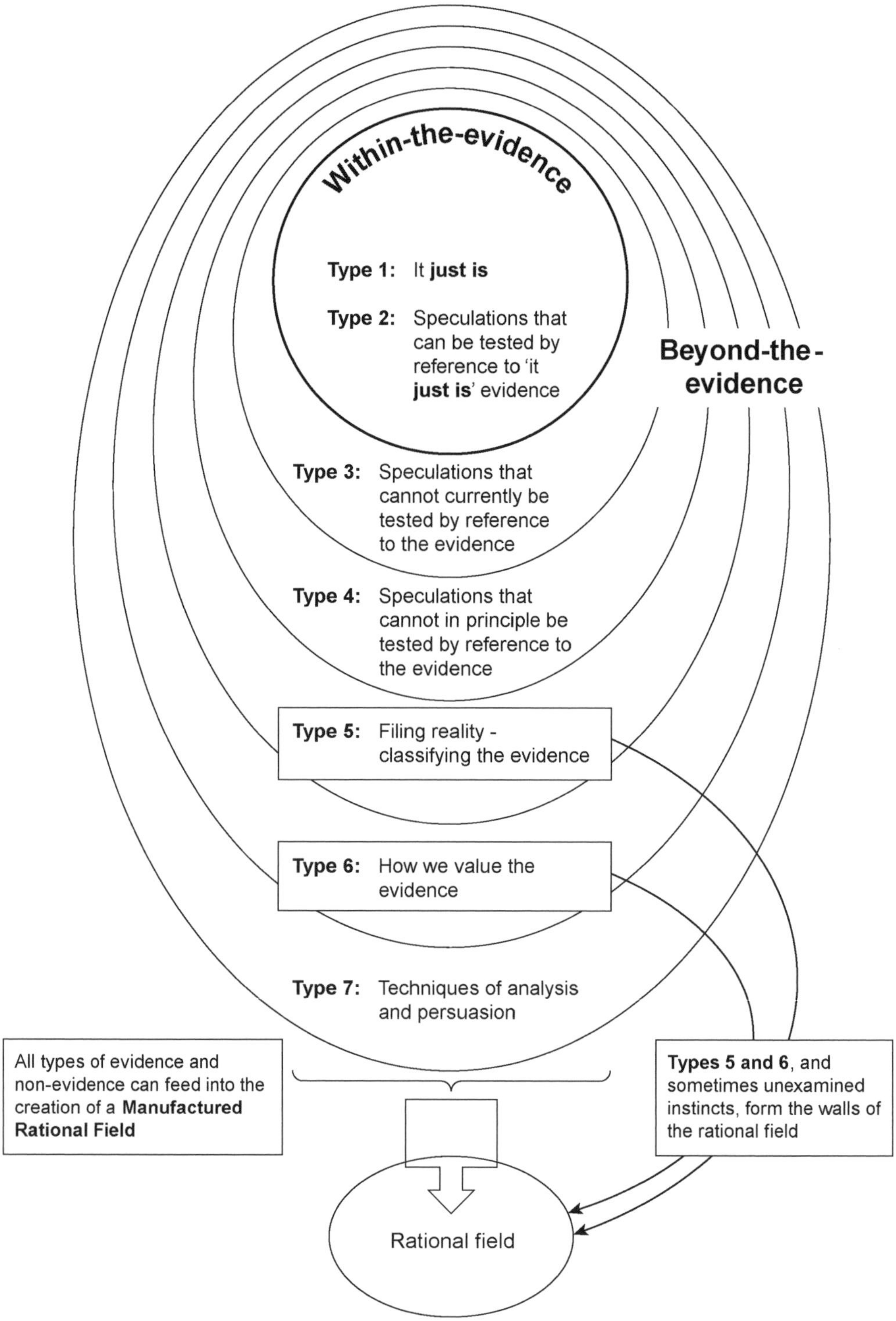

Figure 10 The way in which evidence and non-evidence contribute to the formation of rational fields

source of values). Nonetheless, it is possible to distinguish meaningfully between these categories, as many of the figures in this chapter and **Chapter Six** show.

A manufactured rational field is formed as illustrated in **Figure 10**.

The rational field template – and its formation in beyond-the-evidence is further explained and fully illustrated for use in total health promotion in **Chapter Six**.

The present chapter now explains rational fields in more detail. It concentrates on how to assess the stability of manufactured rational fields, and presents psychiatry and mental health promotion as examples of unstable rational fields. This is important because it develops the argument that psychiatry and mental health promotion are *over-contrived* fields, and it offers ways of assessing the merits – and in particular the internal workings – of existing rational fields. If it can be shown that a rational field is unstable, or disintegrating, this can be a very strong justification for replacing it, or for allowing it to disintegrate without political interference.

THE STABILITY OF RATIONAL FIELDS

A manufactured rational field's stability varies according to the extent to which its goals, strategies and means are clear and coherent, and the extent to which these goals, means and strategies are inspected for clarity and coherence by those within the rational field. A manufactured field's stability also depends on the willingness of those with the power to maintain the field to openly acknowledge and assess the field's forming instincts, classifications and values.

There are four degrees of stability:

1. **Rigid.** A logically consistent field in which all strategies are clearly directed toward the same explicit goal or set of goals. A rigid field cannot respond to changing external circumstances.

2. **Flexible.** A field where not all strategies are fully consistent with each other, and where the field's goal or goals are not completely explicit. A flexible field exhibits some over-simplifications and over-complications of meaning and purpose. A flexible field is able to evolve as circumstances change.

3. **Disintegrating.** A field where some behaviours conflict with each other, and where the field's goal or goals are vague (as they must be to accommodate the conflicts). A disintegrating field exhibits multiple over-simplifications, over-complications and contradictions of meaning and purpose. There are increasing examples of out of context, one-off problem-solving.

4. **Disintegrated.** A field exhibiting so many over-simplifications, over-complications and contradictions of meaning and purpose that its structure has collapsed. There are so many out of context, one-off problem-solving behaviours that new rational fields begin to form.

Note three further points:

First, although rigid rational fields tend to be the most explicit of manufactured rational fields, they are not necessarily the most desirable type. Flexible rational fields tend to be better suited to the differences of interpretation, emphasis and interest involved in real-world decision-making – we humans seem to prefer at least some things to be fudged.

Second, the stability of a field is irrelevant to its moral status: only its content matters with respect to ethics. Teams of charity workers and ruthless invading armies may inhabit equally rigid manufactured rational fields.

Third, over-simplifications and over-complications of classification are the most informative features of manufactured rational fields since they indicate a field's intrinsic stability. Knowing them may also help reveal the strength and extent of the values and classifications that surround any manufactured field.

EXAMPLES OF RATIONAL FIELDS WITH VARIOUS LEVELS OF STABILITY

With one exception (see **Figure 30**, below) all the rational fields discussed in the remainder of this book are manufactured. Here are some simple examples, the most stable first.

A rigid rational field

This simple field (**Figure 11**) has one goal (**Goal X**), toward which both its strategies are aimed.

A flexible rational field

This field (**Figure 12**) is flexible because its goals are not completely explicit, it contains over-simplifications and over-complications of meaning, and not all its behaviours are necessarily consistent with each other.

The goals – to promote health and well-being – seem clear enough at first sight. However, even though many health promoters understand these expressions in similar ways, health and well-being have a range of meanings not fully spelled out in the above field. These meanings are not all harmonious, and not all health promoters favour the same meanings. Furthermore, some of the field's strategies may interfere with or even counteract others within the field. For example, activity to encourage weight loss might conflict with activity to encourage stress-free relaxation (the former might engender guilt in people attempting the latter).

A disintegrating rational field

This field (**Figure 13**) is disintegrating because it contains conflicting strategies directed at incompatible goals. There is also an example of one-off problem-solving within this

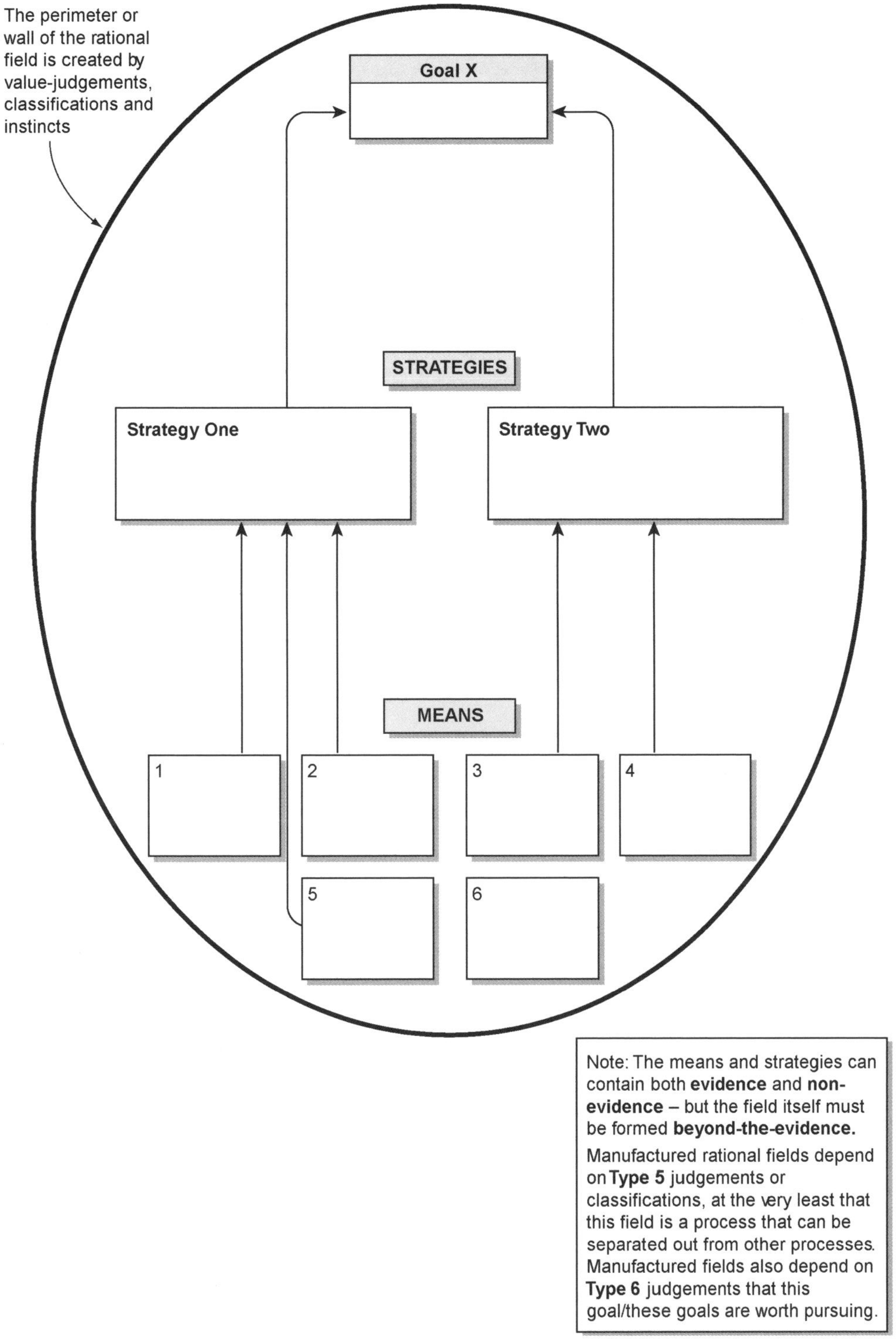
The perimeter or wall of the rational field is created by value-judgements, classifications and instincts
Goal X
STRATEGIES
Strategy One
Strategy Two
MEANS
1
2
3
4
5
6
Note: The means and strategies can contain both **evidence** and **non-evidence** – but the field itself must be formed **beyond-the-evidence.**
Manufactured rational fields depend on **Type 5** judgements or classifications, at the very least that this field is a process that can be separated out from other processes. Manufactured fields also depend on **Type 6** judgements that this goal/these goals are worth pursuing.

Figure 11 A rigid manufactured rational field in the abstract

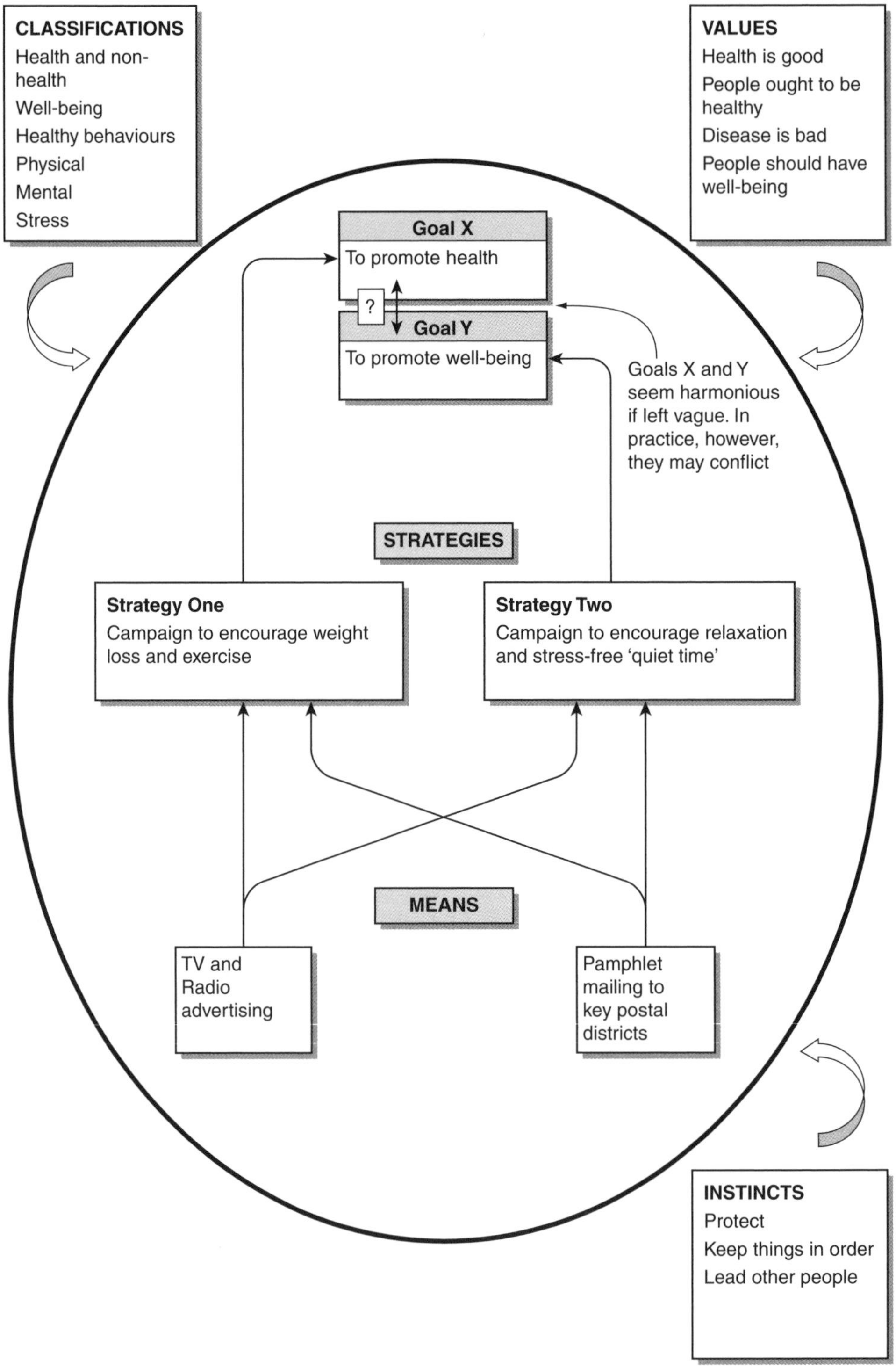

Figure 12 A flexible manufactured rational field (simplified for illustrative purposes)

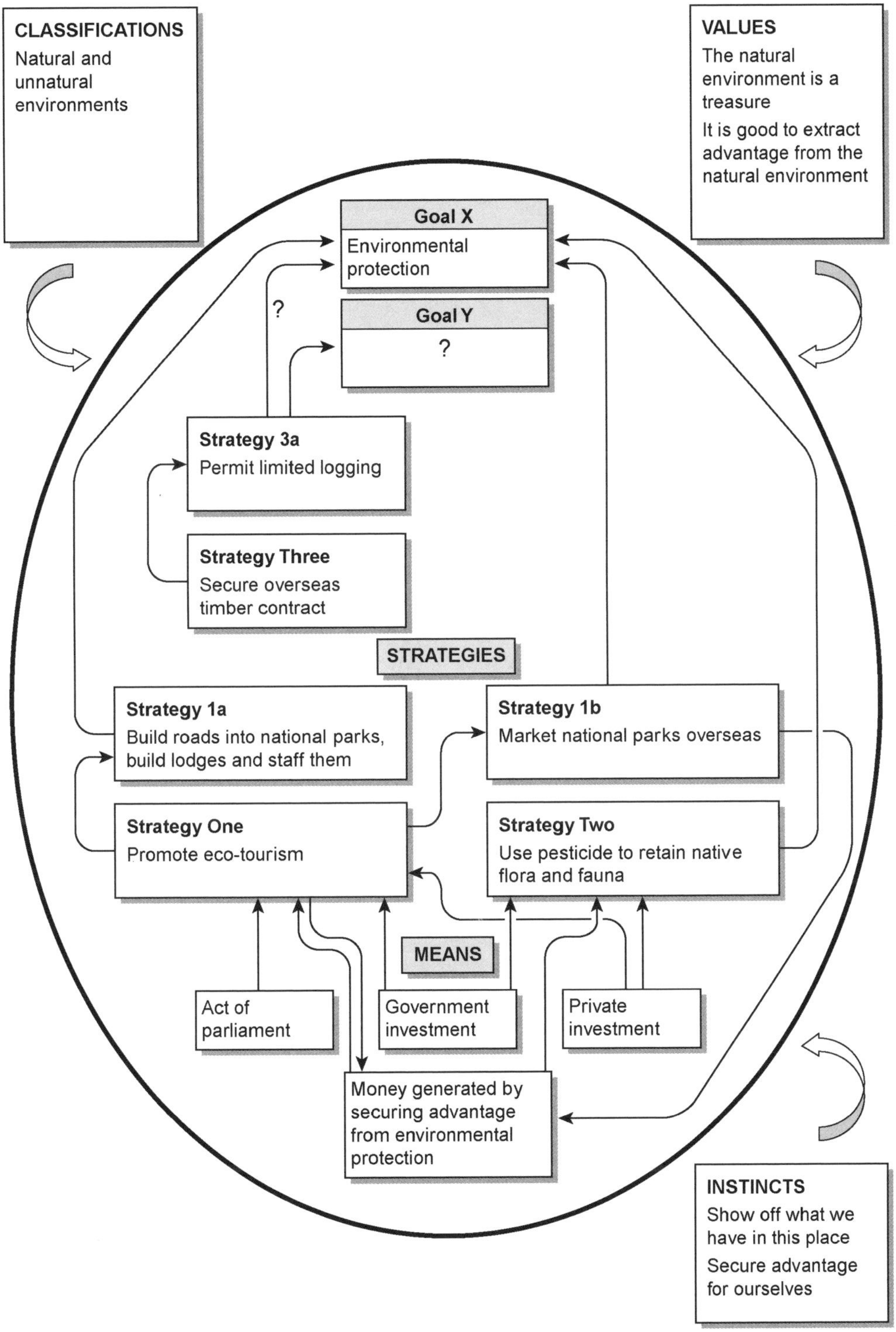

Figure 13 A simple illustrative example of a disintegrating manufactured rational field

field, permitting limited logging of native wood in order to benefit from a lucrative overseas contract.

Most actors in a disintegrating field assume that, despite the conflicts, the different strategies are nevertheless (somehow) all aimed at a coherent goal or at a set of compatible goals. Yet in fact the only reasons conflicting behaviours are possible is because **Goal X** (in this case 'environmental protection') is so vaguely defined, and because the field-generating values, classifications and instincts are left unexamined.

Environmental protection has many different meanings. It can mean 'protecting unadulterated nature' to the naturalist, 'sensitively managing the environment' to government, and even 'naturally enhancing the environment to generate profit' to some business people: some theme park managers, for example, argue that without the funds their parks generate the environment would deteriorate, or would be used for some worse purpose.

A disintegrated rational field

Goals left so vague as to 'justify' conflicting strategies must eventually disintegrate into new rigid rational fields (unless powerful interest groups intervene to preserve the original field by reinforcing its walls of value and classification – in which case a field can persist even if it is overtly irrational, as we shall see). For example, **Figure 14** shows an inexorable progression from **Figure 13**. The competing strategies all said to protect the environment have developed to such an extent that it becomes obvious that they are directed towards substantially different goals. Once this becomes plain – or impossible for even the most biased interest group to deny – new rational fields must form.

PSYCHIATRY AND MENTAL HEALTH PROMOTION ARE DISINTEGRATING RATIONAL FIELDS

Part One of this book discussed the extent to which both psychiatry and mental health promotion rely on beyond-the-evidence assumptions. The following sections carry the exploration further, showing how psychiatric and mental health promotion rational fields may be analysed philosophically.

Both psychiatry and mental health promotion are manufactured rational fields. Because of the lack of explicitness about the make-up and walls of both fields, those who inhabit them can find it very hard to see anything wrong with them (they reside happily within the walls of the field, and cannot see over them). Less partial observers are in a stronger position – from outside the walls it is not difficult to see these rational fields for what they are.

Psychiatry is a disintegrating rational field held together by political force. Mental health promotion is also beginning to disintegrate, despite its relative youth. Both fields' goals tend to be vague and to contain multiple over-simplifications and over-complications of meaning. Rational behaviours within each field are not always consistent with each other and – certainly in the case of psychiatry – there are glaring examples of conflict of both purpose and strategy.

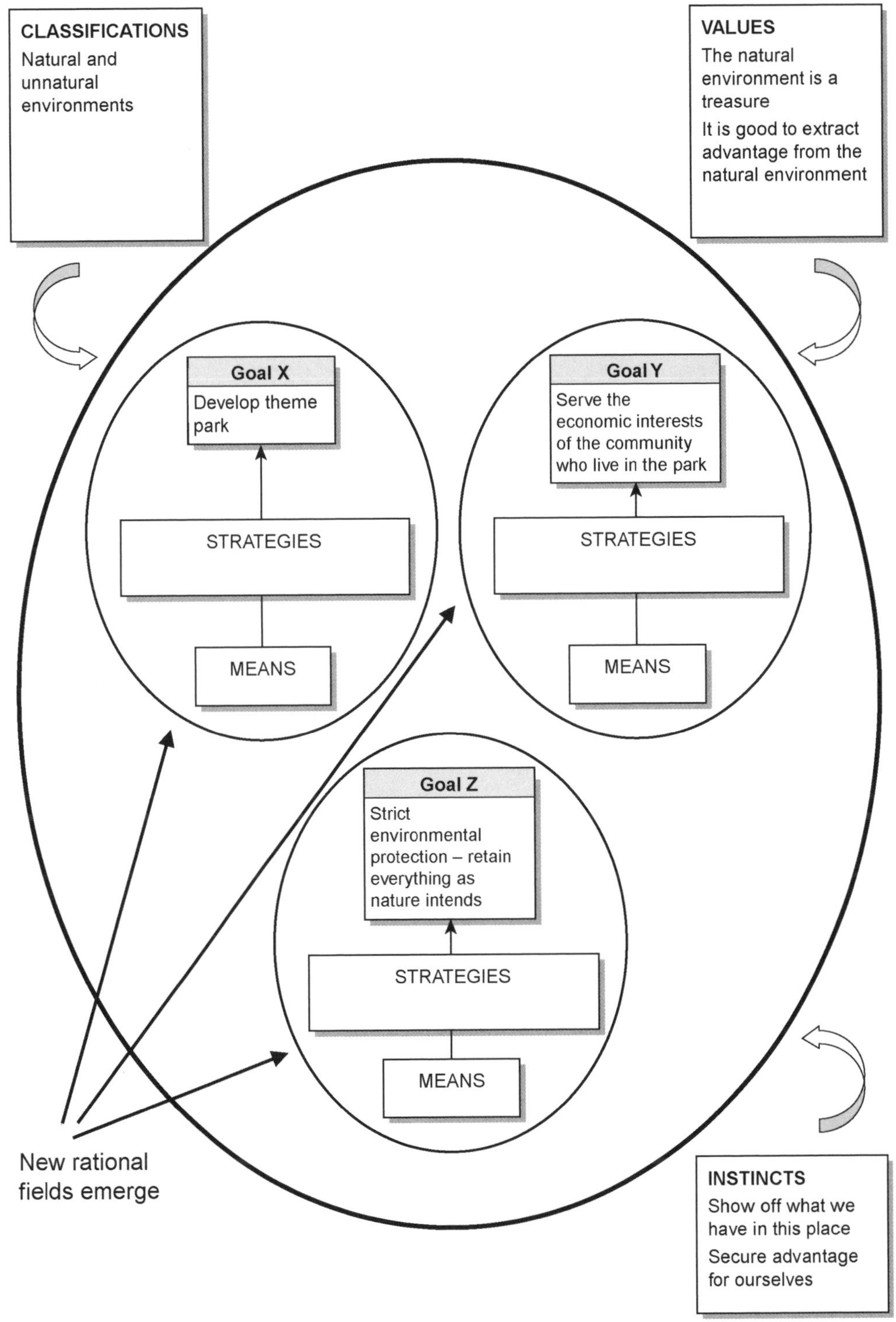

Figure 14 A simple illustrative example of a disintegrated manufactured rational field

CENTRAL PROBLEMS OF CLASSIFICATION AND VALUE

Rational fields disintegrate either because their founding classifications, values and instincts are not recognised, or because their classification system is over-artificial, or both. All the difficulties of the psychiatry and mental health promotion rational fields are caused by such errors. In particular:

Errors of Classification, Value and Logic

Error 1. Using a single term to describe different states and processes

Error 2. Acting as if a particular rational field is the only option, or acting as if only it is true and all others are false

Error 3. Using different terms to describe states and processes that are fundamentally identical

Error 4. Knowingly constructing artificial divisions within or between rational fields

Error 5. Creating over-elaborate rational fields

Error 6. Not noticing or disregarding beyond-the-evidence decisions and assumptions

Error 7. Failing to provide comprehensive explanations and justifications of the value-judgements and instincts that make up the perimeter of the field

Error 8. Perpetuating rational fields that incorporate contradictory notions

CENTRAL ERRORS OF CLASSIFICATION, VALUE AND LOGIC IN PSYCHIATRY AND MENTAL HEALTH PROMOTION'S RATIONAL FIELDS

Error 1. Using a single term to describe different states and processes

Error 1 occurs when single terms are continually used to represent conceptually distinct ideas. For example, in psychiatry 'mental illness' is repeatedly allowed to stand for 'brain disorder', 'disorder of the mind', 'lack of insight', 'depression', 'injury', 'personality disorder' and myriad other terms, even though these expressions are not the same. In mental health promotion, 'mental health' is used to stand for concepts like 'optimism', 'resilience', 'happiness' and 'well-being', each of which can also have different meanings.

Some of this over-simplification is inevitable, and not a problem. 'I work for mental health' or 'I treat mental illness' is often sufficient information in casual conversation.

Nor is it a problem if the general term is defined more specifically – 'I specialise in the treatment of certain kinds of psychosis', for instance. However, over-simplification is a problem if it disguises substantial questions. For example, if the term 'mental illness' is habitually used to represent both 'brain disorder' and 'disorder of the mind' then exploration of the possible differences between these states is effectively prohibited.

Does the fact that a person feels sad and anxious mean she must have a brain disorder? Is it possible to treat a disorder of the mind by chemical therapies? These are important questions. Careful thought about the meaning of words is required to answer them. To say they are all aspects of mental health or mental illness, and automatically to deal with them in conventional ways, is to ignore central and unresolved issues in the psychiatric rational field.

The American Psychiatric Association's (APA) *Diagnostic and Statistical Manual of Mental Disorders, Volume IV* offers a striking example of **Error 1**, at p. xxi. It confesses:

> ...although this manual provides a classification of mental disorders, it must be admitted that no definition adequately specifies precise boundaries for the concept of mental disorder.[54]

Not defining the centremost term in psychiatry protects psychiatric work behind a verbal smog. Of course, from the point of view of the APA, not only is this acceptable, it is necessary. Serious internal debate about the nature of mental disorder would inevitably bring other tenets of the profession into question: if mental disorder is a vague idea then so are schizophrenia, personality disorder and dissociation, for example. The APA cannot entertain extensive analysis of mental disorder because this would explicitly propel the psychiatric field into disintegration.

The same is true of mental health promotion, where the situation can be pictured as shown in **Figure 15**.

Error 2. Acting as if a particular rational field is the only option, or acting as if only it is true and all others are false

One of the consequences of setting up systems to interpret the world is that they tend to exclude incompatible systems. For example, psychiatry cannot encompass the idea of demonic possession because this is not specified as an illness within the psychiatric field. Equally, personal illness theory, which holds that 'mental illness': '...refers primarily to an adverse change in the ability to relate to other persons and in the ability to intend one's own actions'[106] is incompatible with the conventional psychiatric field because it cannot encompass the idea that schizophrenia is a specific disease entity.[107] In turn, most indigenous people's understandings of the world cannot accommodate the idea that mental illness is something separate from a person's being in the world:

> ...for Aboriginal people health and sickness are often understood in terms of relationships between people.[108]

If this diversity of interpretation is recognised and valued – if rational fields are treated as speculations, as stabs at defining and negotiating reality – then it is possible to use them constructively, if circumstances require it. We cannot escape rational fields – we are both enabled and restricted by them – and we must create at least one rational field if we are to make any choices at all. The challenge is to create or inhabit

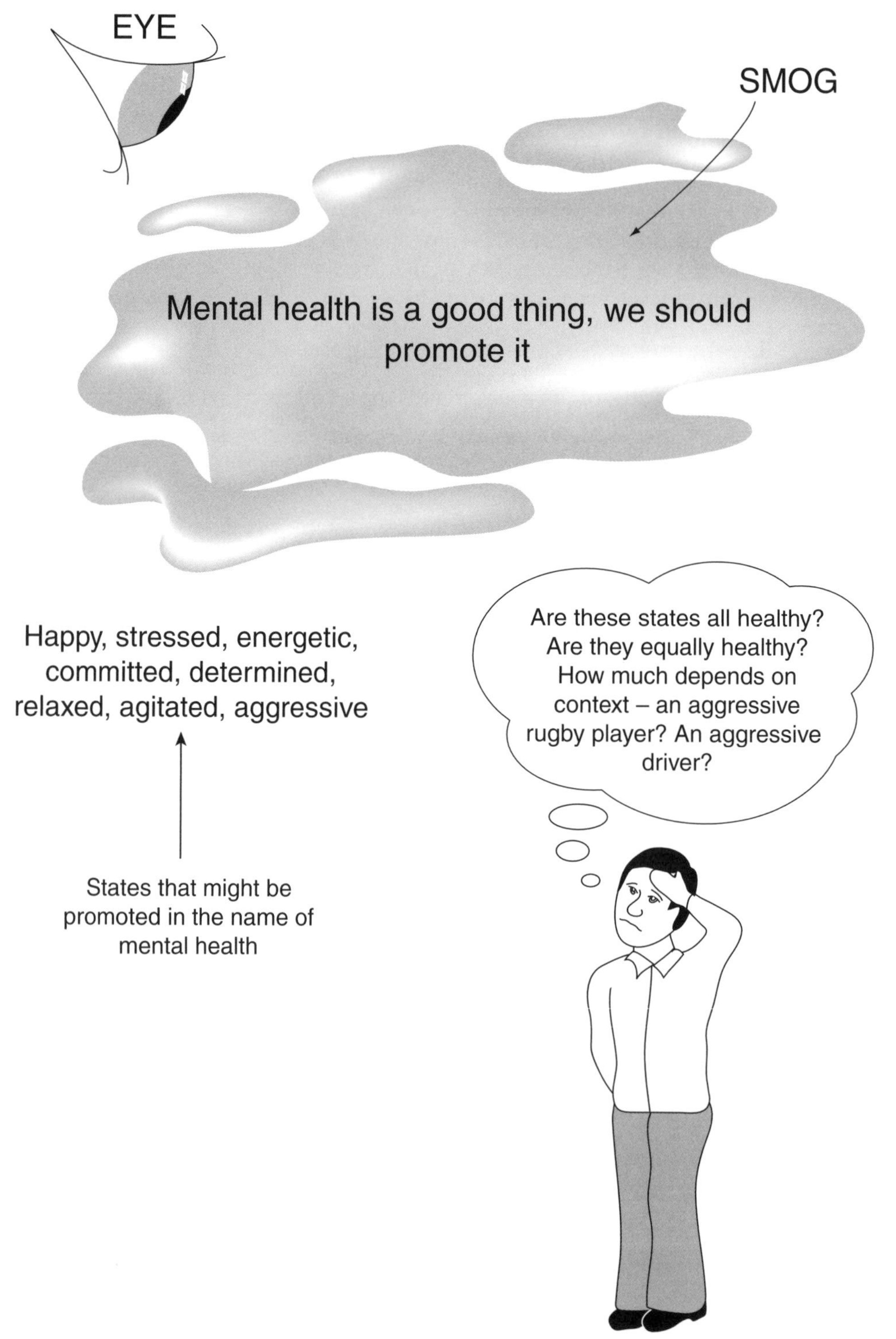
EYE
SMOG
Mental health is a good thing, we should promote it
Happy, stressed, energetic, committed, determined, relaxed, agitated, aggressive
States that might be promoted in the name of mental health
Are these states all healthy? Are they equally healthy? How much depends on context – an aggressive rugby player? An aggressive driver?

Figure 15 Error 1 in mental health promotion

rational fields that have sufficient flexibility to allow us to assess the value of other fields – and to move in and out of them if we wish.

If the fields we live in are too rigid or over-flexible our understanding of the world and our problem-solving abilities become dramatically inhibited.[109] Actually to advocate one rational field to the exclusion of all others is worse still. As we saw in **Chapter Two**, the psychiatric profession repeatedly engages in an aggressive/defensive advocacy of its rational field. As a result its disciples understand and care very little about the ways alternative systems attempt to deal with the problems of human experience.[110]

Error 3. Using different terms to describe states and processes that are fundamentally identical

Error 3 – the reverse of **Error 1** – occurs when words meant to stand for different states and processes are used to describe phenomena with a single basic essence. For example, in psychiatry labels such as 'illness', 'disease', 'disorder', 'insanity', 'sickness', 'malfunction', 'chemical imbalance', 'schizophrenia', 'bi-polar disorder' and so on, are used to discriminate states of reality. This incessant differentiation makes it look as if these terms describe unique entities, different from other entities in all respects. Yet so long as the different terms describe problems of living (which they are bound to in psychiatry) they will always and essentially indicate *losses of autonomy*.[111,112]

Mental health promoters commonly use terms like 'being well', 'recovering','adapting' and 'having positive health'. Just like the psychiatric labels, their repeated use makes it appear as if they are different states, and yet at bottom each describes a situation that is essentially *the exercise of autonomy*.

In either context, the effect of using different terms to describe the same basic state is to mask work for health under a verbal blizzard. In the case of psychiatry the situation might be pictured as in **Figure 16**.

In order to help people move forward it is necessary to use different words to specify the type of deficit in autonomy (or health) they are suffering from. For example, being unable to speak at social gatherings is a different problem from having grandiose ideas: muteness in company will require a different linguistic explanation and most probably a different therapy from a delusion of grandeur. However, it is one thing to use special terms to describe different manifestations of loss of autonomy. And quite another to see only a flurry of categories, each with a meaning separate from other meanings, existing within a rational field you think of as the only plausible interpretation of reality.

Error 4. Knowingly constructing artificial divisions within or between rational fields

Error 4 occurs when helpful conceptual clarifications are confused with proofs that reality is one way rather than any other (this is very obviously a **Type 5** beyond-the-evidence error).

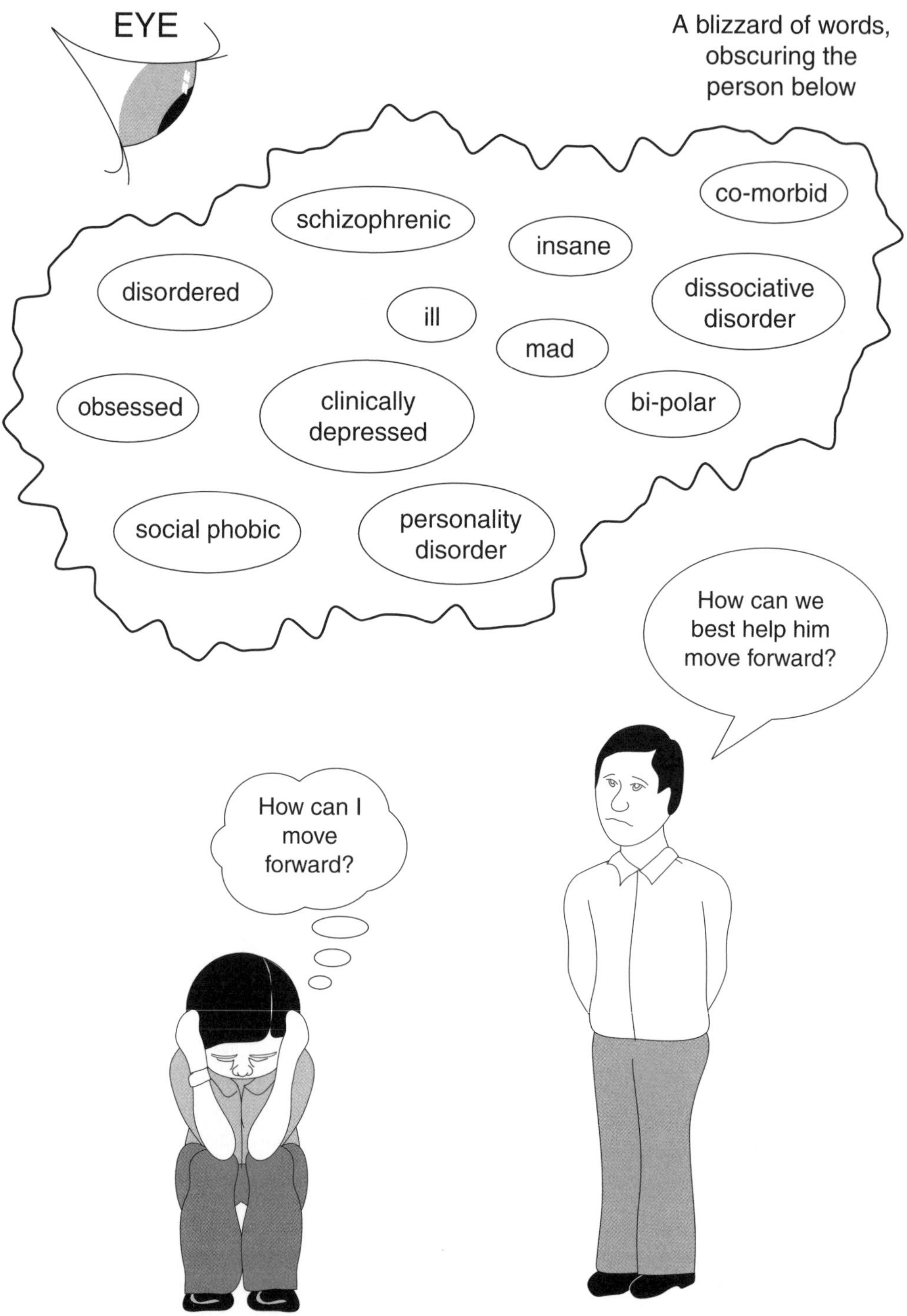

Figure 16 Error 3 in psychiatry

Mental illness ----------------|---------------- **Mental health**
(meaning: no mental health) (meaning: no mental illness)

Figure 17 Mental illness and mental health conceived of as opposites

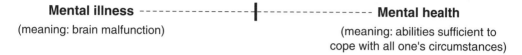

Mental illness ----------------|---------------- **Mental health**
(meaning: brain malfunction) (meaning: abilities sufficient to cope with all one's circumstances)

Figure 18 The poles defined in a non-mutually exclusive way

Mental health promotion is particularly prone to this form of over-complication. Some mental health promotion theorists attempt conceptual clarification in order to better understand the purpose and scope of their field.[113,114] They are right to do so, and set a good example for the psychiatrists. But unfortunately problems arise when the results of their philosophical explorations are considered to be **just is** discoveries – discoveries about the world as it is – rather than beyond-the-evidence classifications, which is what they really are.

The clearest example of **Error 4** can be seen in the now standard mental health promotion argument that the psychiatric understanding of mental health erroneously links mental health and mental illness. The argument goes like this.

If mental health and illness are thought of as logical opposites, the spectrum illustrated in **Figure 17** is sufficient to describe their relationship.

However, if the poles of the continuum are defined in a non-mutually exclusive way, for instance as in **Figure 18** a move toward one pole might pull the pointer away from the other, but will not necessarily do so. For example, a decrease in a person's ability to cope may or may not imply deteriorating brain function.

These poles are impossible to represent on a single continuum. Consequently, mental health promoters advocate dual continua. Thus, the mental health pole of **Figure 18** might become a continuum in its own right, as shown in **Figure 19**. And the mental illness pole might become as **Figure 20**.

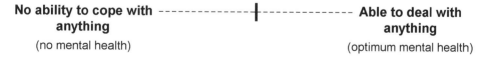

No ability to cope with anything -------------|------------- **Able to deal with anything**
(no mental health) (optimum mental health)

Figure 19 A mental health spectrum

Total brain malfunction ------------|------------ **Normal brain function**
(total mental illness) (no mental illness)

Figure 20 A mental illness spectrum

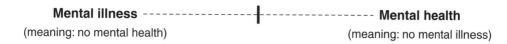

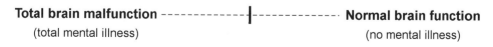

Severe brain malfunction -----|--------------------- **Normal brain function**
(severe mental illness) (no mental illness)

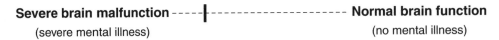

Figure 21 Another mental illness spectrum

No ability to cope with anything ---------------------|----- **Competent to deal with all prevailing circumstances**
(no mental health) (optimum mental health)

Figure 22 Another mental health spectrum

These (and other) dual continua establish the conceptual flexibility to disconnect mental illness and mental health. For example, a person might have a brain malfunction that places her well to the left on the mental illness spectrum, as depicted in **Figure 21** and yet – if she lives with a supportive family, or has learnt techniques to deal creatively with her brain problem – she could be well to the right on the mental health continuum, as shown in **Figure 22**.

Equally, a person could have normal brain function (and so sit at the absolute right of the mental illness spectrum) and yet at the same time be in circumstances so inappropriate to his abilities that he is forced to the left of the 'mental health' continuum – if he is a long-term unemployed person unable to find work, or if he is a colonised and displaced aborigine, for example.[115]

Seen in one way this use of dual continua liberates. There is plainly more to promoting mental health than tackling mental illness. However, the problem is that this separation of continua creates division – it manufactures two separate fields when there need be only one, based on the goal to create autonomy.

It does not follow from the use of a technique to demonstrate a difference between psychiatric goals and more broadly focused health goals that psychiatry and mental health promotion are actually incommensurable endeavours. Unfortunately, **Error 4** creates the perfect environment for unhelpful competition between psychiatry and mental health promotion (in the process causing endless and pointless disputes between rival factions[55]).

Error 5. Creating over-elaborate rational fields

Particularly in psychiatry, continuing revision and expansion of diagnostic categories has created a blizzard of diseases and illnesses and their sub-types so thick and fierce that it sometimes obscures everything human about the person (or persons) so classified. For example:

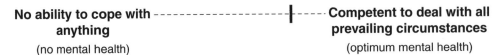

> **Bipolar I Disorder** is distinguished from **Major Depressive Disorder** and **Dysthymic Disorder** by the lifetime history of at least one **Manic or Mixed Episode**. **Bipolar I Disorder** is distinguished from **Bipolar II Disorder** by the presence of one or more **Manic or Mixed Episodes**. When an individual previously diagnosed with **Bipolar II Disorder** develops a **Manic or Mixed Episode**, the diagnosis is changed to **Bipolar I Disorder**.

> In **Cyclothymic Disorder**, there are numerous periods of hypomanic symptoms that do not meet criteria for a **Manic Episode** and periods of depressive symptoms that do not meet symptom or duration criteria for a **Major Depressive Episode**. **Bipolar I Disorder** is distinguished from **Cyclothymic Disorder** by the presence of one or more **Manic Or Mixed Episodes**. If a **Manic or Mixed Episode** occurs after the first 2 years of **Cyclothymic Disorder**, then **Cyclothymic Disorder** and **Bipolar I Disorder** may both be diagnosed.
>
> The differential diagnosis between **Psychotic disorders** (e.g., **Schizoaffective Disorder**, **Schizophrenia**, and **Delusional Disorder**) and **Bipolar I Disorder** may be difficult (especially in adolescents) because these disorders may share a number of presenting symptoms (e.g., grandiose and persecutory delusions, irritability, agitation, and catatonic symptoms), particularly cross-sectionally and early in their course... Manic and depressive symptoms may be present during **Schizophrenia**, **Delusional Disorder**, and **Psychotic Disorder Not Otherwise Specified**, but rarely with sufficient number, duration, and pervasiveness to meet criteria for a **Manic Episode** or a **Major Depressive Episode**. However, when full criteria are met (or the symptoms are of particular clinical significance), a diagnosis of **Bipolar Disorder Not Otherwise Specified** may be made in addition to the diagnosis of **Schizophrenia**, **Delusional Disorder**, or **Psychotic Disorder Not Otherwise Specified**.
>
> If there is a very rapid alternation (over days) between manic symptoms and depressive symptoms (e.g., several days of purely manic symptoms followed by several days of purely depressive symptoms) that do not meet minimal duration criteria for a **Manic Episode** or **Major Depressive Episode**, the diagnosis is **Bipolar Disorder Not Otherwise Specified**.[116]

There are psychiatrists who believe these distinctions are real. From within psychiatry's rational field they probably look real. However, from outside the field they look ludicrously artificial. They are almost laughable. For example, in the above quote the DSM-IV states that: '**Bipolar I Disorder** is distinguished from **Cyclothymic Disorder** by the presence of one or more **Manic Or Mixed Episodes**.' However: 'If a **Manic or Mixed Episode** occurs after the first 2 years of **Cyclothymic Disorder**, then **Cyclothymic Disorder** and **Bipolar I Disorder** may both be diagnosed.' It is hard not to see this as absurd. Psychiatrists are told that the distinguishing feature of cyclothymic disorder is no 'manic or mixed episodes'. But after two years (why two years? Why not 23 months or 25 months or four years?) a 'manic or mixed episode' can confirm cyclothymic disorder.

It is also possible to diagnose both **Bipolar II Disorder** and **Cyclothymic Disorder** if there are **Major Depressive Episodes** after two years, and yet in the first two years there can be no **Manic or Mixed Episodes** or **Major Depressive Episodes**. It is not clear (to me at least) what magical change occurs after two years in a patient with **Cyclothymic Disorder** sufficient to justify symptoms meaning he is not **Cyclothymic** for the first 730 days meaning exactly the opposite from day 731 onwards.

It has been repeatedly demonstrated[117] that the more categories and sub-categories invented the more difficult it is to decide between them:

> ...Bleuler[118] claimed that all the symptoms of manic-depressive psychosis may occur in schizophrenia. Without some hierarchical notion, how does one decide which of the clusters of symptoms is so dominant as to warrant making one diagnosis rather than the other? There are no public rules. Each clinician is left to his own subjective devices.[119]

Furthermore, not all psychiatrists subscribe to the American Psychiatric Association's classification system. For example, as noted earlier, Foulds has argued for an alternative way of classifying mental illness. He calls his system the 'hierarchy of personal illness'. He says:

> The personal illness model is concerned... to restore person-hood, that is to restore the ability to enter into mutual, personal relationships and the ability to intend one's own actions.
>
> The medical model is essentially concerned with illness of the organism in the sense of 'that which we have in common with the animals'. The aim is to restore the normal functioning of the organism.[120]

The personal illness model has fewer categories than the psychiatric or medical one. Unsurprisingly, when he used it to diagnose patients, Foulds found it simpler. In particular, in a study of 480 patients, he found it considerably reduced the incidence of 'overlap of symptoms':

> The results indicate that 58% of 480 psychiatric patients fell into only one syndrome within the class to which they were finally assigned, when the hierarchy of classes of personal illness was used; when the hierarchy was not used, the percentage of unmixed syndromes fell to a mere 13%. It is, therefore, quite clear that... psychiatric diagnosis is of no value because there is too much overlap between syndromes...[121]

In other words, a simpler system produces less overlap between symptoms and therefore renders diagnoses more plausible.

The more unnecessarily complex the system, the more unstable the rational field.

Error 6. Not noticing or disregarding beyond-the-evidence decisions and assumptions

Manufactured rational fields are formed by instincts or by favouring some values ahead of others. It is impossible for any rational field to justify these founding values by reference to its internal goals. However logical it is, no field can answer the question 'why is Goal X worth pursuing?' without reference to a belief external to the system.

Most actors within most rational fields never notice this (they simply proceed within the norms of whatever established rational field they inhabit). Yet it ought to be blindingly obvious since it is a law of the social realm that:

Various Pieces of Evidence + Various Sorts of Opinion = a Plan of Action

Both evidence and opinion are required to create a plan.[63] If you have an opinion and no evidence, at best you have an hypothesis rather than a plan. And if you don't have an opinion then you cannot choose between the multitude of evidence that surrounds you (you cannot possibly have a plan without an opinion).

A geneticist's plan to clone a sheep and my daughter's plan to persuade me to let her have a third piece of chocolate both conform to the above formula – evidence is needed (of genetic mechanisms, of what strategies usually work for my daughter to twist me round her little finger) but opinion is also necessary (and necessary first) to interpret and select from the evidence (it is good to clone a sheep, it is a social priority to clone a sheep, I desire more chocolate, I must have another Freddo bar).

Error 7. Failing to provide comprehensive explanations and justifications of the value-judgements and instincts that make up the perimeter of the field

If you do not state the reason *why* something is being done and instead concentrate only on how to do it then things can look misleadingly simple – the only challenge seems to be to achieve the task in hand, as efficiently as possible within the closed field. All your thinking is done within a rational field (within walls created from beyond-the-evidence). None of your thinking is done *about* the rational field itself. In other words you ignore beyond-the-evidence **Types 5** and **6**. And this means that you do not have to worry whether your tasks make sense when viewed from outside the field, you do not have to worry whether your tasks are moral or reasonable so long as they are allowed within the field, and you do not even have to worry whether they are the best choices out of all the other tasks you might be doing outside the field's perimeter – rather you just get on and do whatever is justified by your manufactured rational field.

An Example

Here is a pertinent example. Several million children (around 5 million in the USA alone[110]) are being treated with Ritalin (methylphenidate) and other stimulants on the ground that they have attention deficit-hyperactivity disorder (ADHD) – or just plain attention deficit disorder (ADD) – and suffer from inattention, hyperactivity, or 'impulsivity'. Within a closed rational system this can make sense. It presumably makes perfect sense to those psychiatrists who prescribe Ritalin to children (see **Figure 23**).

It is possible to incorporate some 'disbenefits' in the internal calculations within a flexible rational field (for example, withdrawal from Ritalin can sometimes cause depression, exhaustion, physiological abnormalities, suicide and other psychiatric disturbances[110]). However, since Ritalin apparently does calm children down and make them more manageable these 'disbenefits' are outweighed – at least within the rational field depicted in **Figure 23** – by the achievement of Goals X and Y.

The field in this figure depends on both evidence (certain behaviours happen, Ritalin has an effect on these behaviours) and classifications and values (ADHD is a mental illness, children ought to concentrate at school). These opinions lie behind the choice of Goals X and Y, but they are not justified by the rational field itself, and are of course not justified by the evidence alone either.

If those inside the field do not examine its perimeters they will not appreciate the beyond-the-evidence sources of Goals X and Y. Instead these goals will just seem to be obviously the right thing to do.

Furthermore, it is impossible (even with the most powerful political influence) within this closed rational field, to incorporate goals based on classifications and values that *conflict fundamentally* with the classifications and values behind Goals X and Y. For example, parent education, curriculum change, and understandings of children's

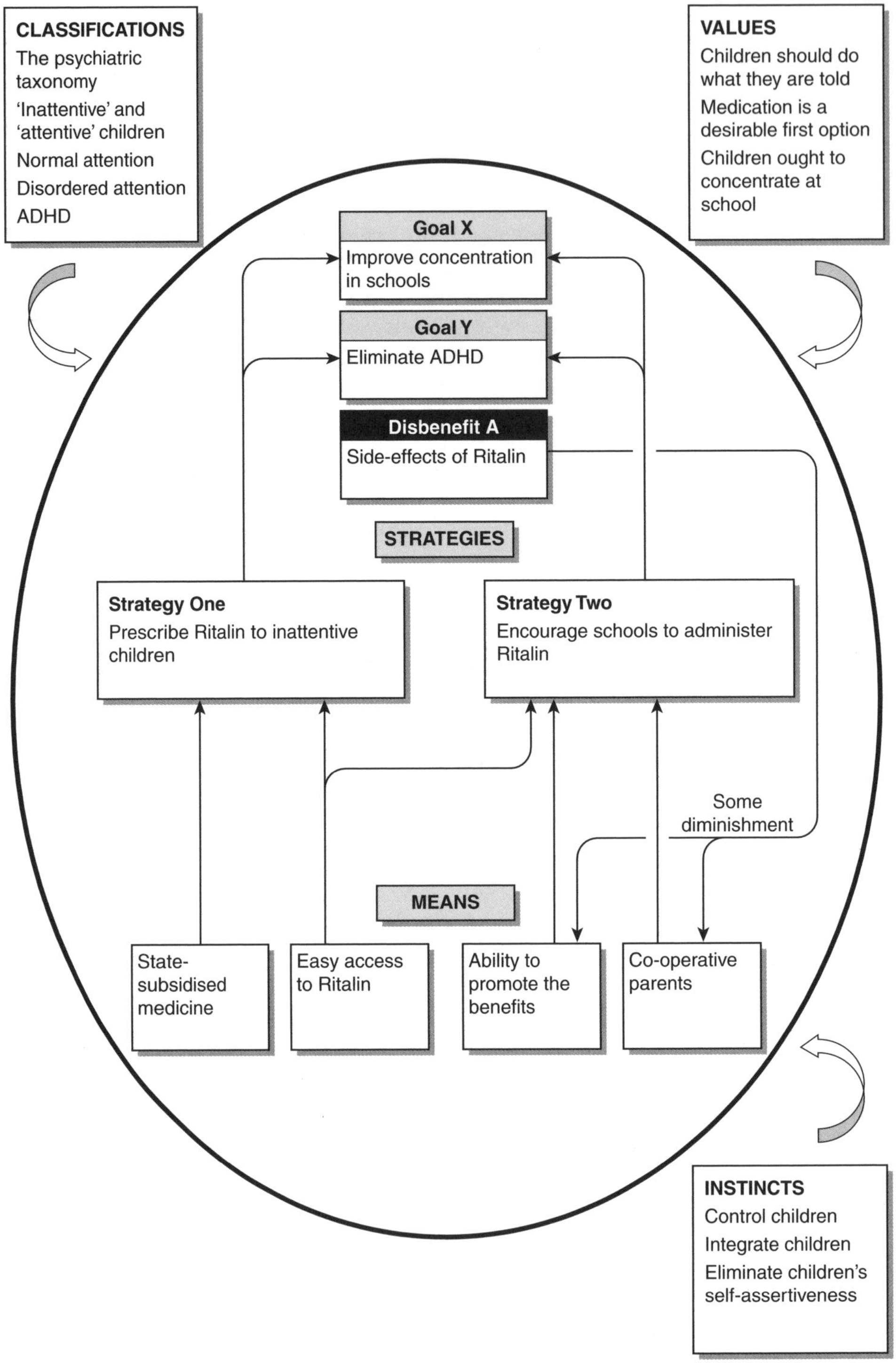

Figure 23 An illustrative closed manufactured rational field (from a conventional psychiatric point of view)

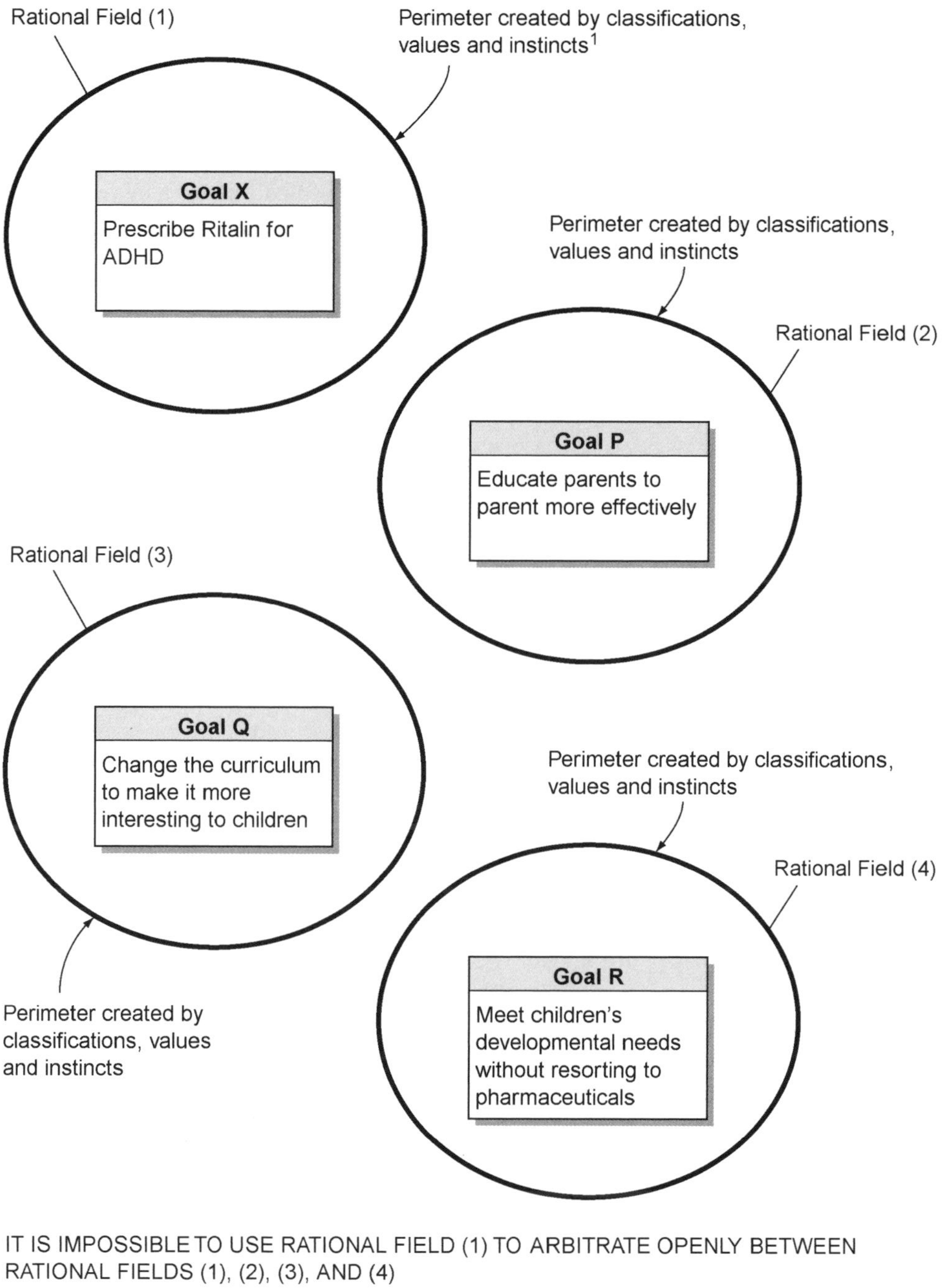

Figure 24 Rational Field 1 instantly becomes questionable when seen alongside alternative rational fields

behaviour which do *not* involve defining them as psychiatrically disordered do not fit within the 'let's prescribe Ritalin' field. The Ritalin field makes sense only when seen from within. But it instantly becomes questionable if it is seen alongside alternative rational fields (see **Figure 24**).

To fail to provide comprehensive explanations and justifications of the classifications, value-judgements and instincts that make up the perimeter of the field is to give the impression that the world is simple and straightforward, when quite the opposite is true. It is also either to deny the presence of values, classifications and instincts at all, or to assume they justify themselves (neither of which is the case).

To try to insert these additional goals within the 'let's prescribe Ritalin' rational field (depicted in **Figure 23**) would create irresolvable conflicts, rendering the field irrational and causing it to disintegrate.

Certainly not everyone is happy about the use of Ritalin to drug active children:

> ADHD (attention deficit hyperactivity disorder) afflicts five percent of the entire student population under eighteen. The symptoms include distractibility, impulsiveness, knee-jiggling, toe-tapping and inability to sit still... books about ADD (attention deficit disorder) are sprouting all over the place... the authors (of one)[122] are committed to the notion that ADD is a neurological condition, genetically transmitted. They elaborate:
>
> > ADD lives in the biology of the brain and the central nervous system. The exact mechanism underlying ADD remains unknown.
>
> ....Yet, apparently, none of the experts on ADD has bothered to investigate the possible school causes of attention deficit disorder...[123]

This is a crucial point and ought to be painfully obvious, and yet it is not obvious if you are smack in the middle of the closed and manufactured 'let's prescribe Ritalin' rational field. Trapped in there, you are chained to the notion that ADD/ADHD is a medical condition, even though you have no idea *how* it is a medical condition – you must be committed to it because you are committed to the rational field, as are the schools and the teachers who administer Ritalin and other stimulants to children every day.

You are not, of course, committed to the view that it might be you, your school and your insightless rational field that is causing the problem by not giving 'distractible children' sufficient structure: within your rational field distractibility must be the problem because the field you are committed to surely cannot itself be the problem. Seen from an alternative rational field – for instance, the field of a committed homeschooler who can advance all manner of reasons why schooling is a damaging institution – the distractibility is a perfectly appropriate response to a social situation that offers nothing constructive to the 'distractible child': within the homeschooler's rational field the school's the problem, not the child.

Error 8. Perpetuating rational fields that incorporate contradictory notions

If rational fields clearly incorporate conflicting goals and methods then they have gone beyond flexibility into disintegration. Left to their own devices they would dissipate into new, initially rigid, rational fields.

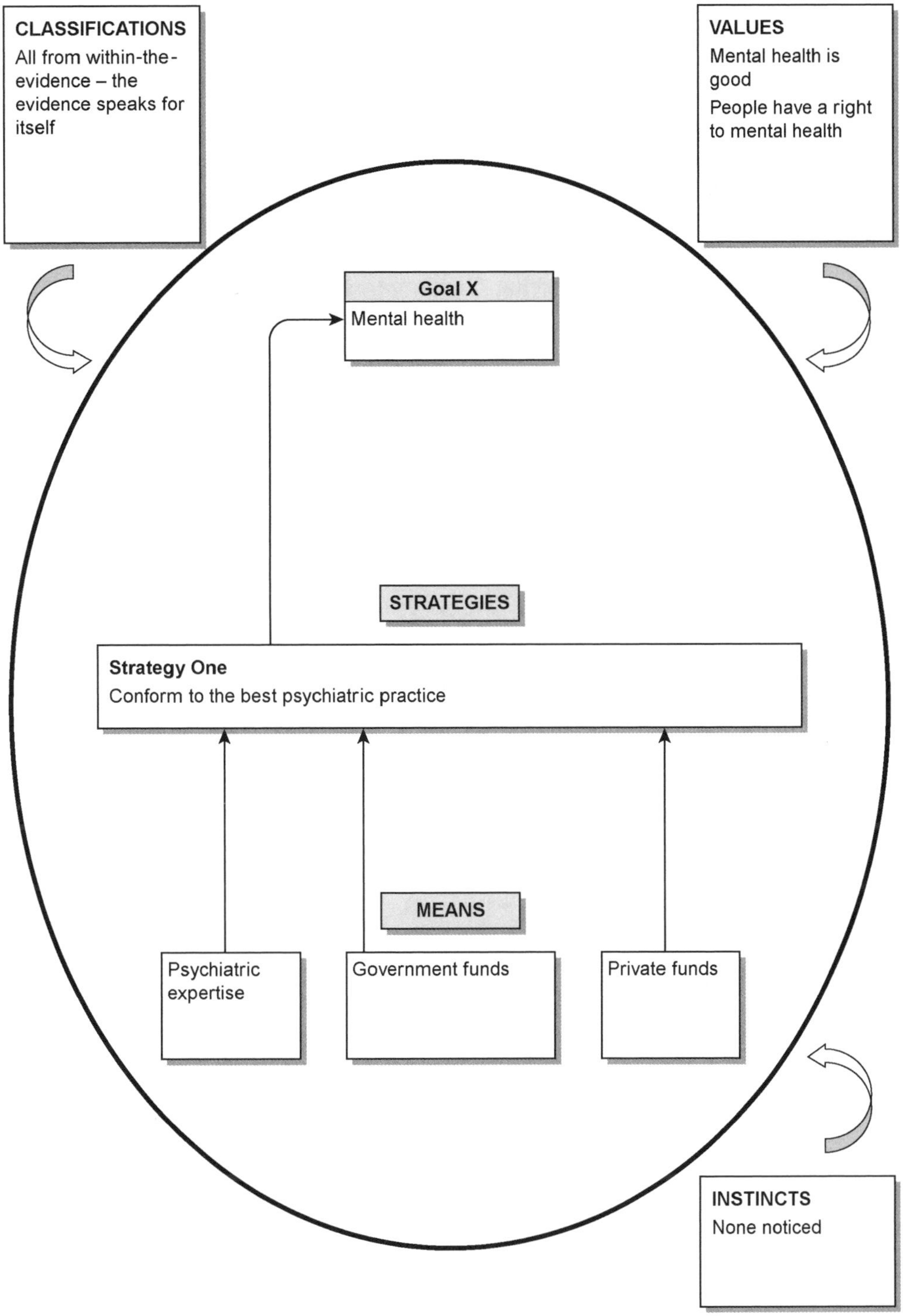

Figure 25 How psychiatry looks to psychiatrists who see it as a unified and harmonious field

This is the case with psychiatry, according to many commentators. It is certainly true that there are major conflicts of goals uneasily contained within the general psychiatric field. For example, there are goals generated by the belief that all psychiatric work should be directed toward recovery of well-being or a meaningful life – regardless of whether or not people are cured of their mental illnesses[124] (this may be called the **Recovery Field)**; there are goals generated by the belief that cure of illness is all that matters[125] (this may be called the **Cure Field)**; and there are also goals (not often admitted to) generated by the view that mentally ill people should be punished for bad behaviours[126] (call this the **Punishment Field**). Each of these goals exists under the general and unexamined (within the rational field) assumption that psychiatry is a unified body of professionals working for the improvement of mental health and to overcome mental disorder.

If gross over-simplification and over-complication of classification is accepted then psychiatry looks like the unified rational field of **Figure 25**. But in harsh reality some of the goals of psychiatry are logically incompatible – i.e. the achievement of one of them renders the achievement of another of them impossible – and yet psychiatry proceeds as if united (see **Figure 26**).

The most simple example (and admittedly this whole idea is simplified) is that there is a fundamental inconsistency between the idea of psychiatry as being to control dangerous people to protect the safety of others (which involves coercion, committal, seclusion, forced treatment and so on *primarily in the interests of safety*) and psychiatry as work to enable their recovery or to care for them (which involves empathy, compassion, empowerment and so on *primarily in the interests of the promotion of autonomy*). It might be argued that sometimes control is necessary in order to move a person into a situation where he can be cared for. However, when control becomes an end in itself – as it sometimes does[126] – then the psychiatric field would simply disintegrate as a consequence of the blatant contradictions, were it not for the exercise of political power and blind faith in established procedures.

RATIONAL FIELDS AND THE FOUNDATIONS THEORY OF HEALTH

If one takes the view (as I do) that it is better that we keep our rational fields as explicit as possible, that we should be continually aware that all rational fields are sustained by values and classifications they cannot justify internally, and that we ought to be able to see alternatives beyond any given rational field at will, then both the current psychiatric and the mental health promotion fields should be abandoned. They should be replaced by a single, explicitly health-promoting field, governed by the understanding that promoting a person's health means promoting the autonomy of an integrated being in a social context – promoting the autonomy of a human rational field (a person) amongst countless other rational fields, in a way that can incorporate other understandings and approaches so long as they contribute to the promotion of health.

The field should be flexible, but not so flexible that it flirts with disintegration. Disintegration can be avoided if all the actors in it understand its philosophical basis – that

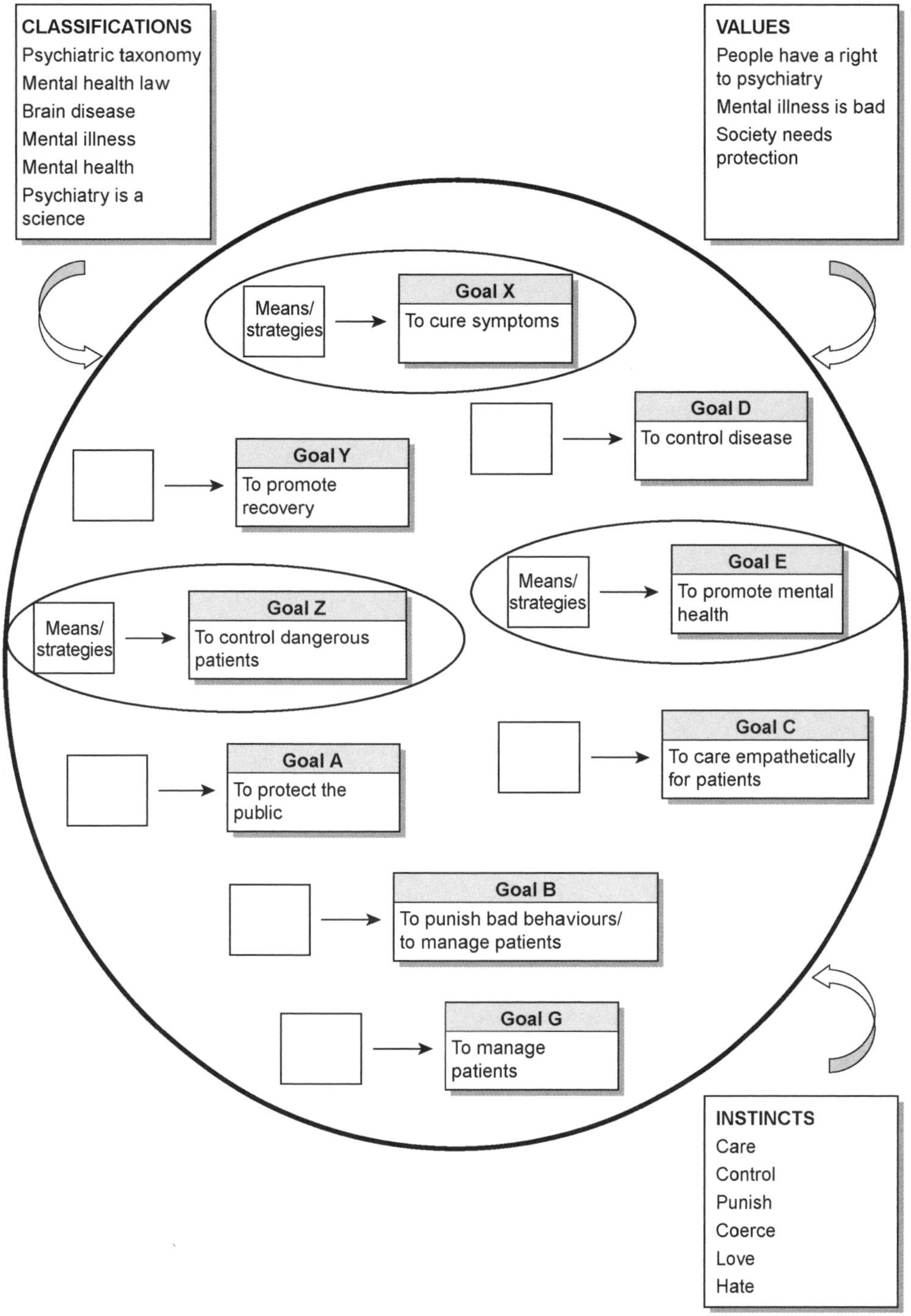

Figure 26 Multiple manufactured rational fields uneasily held together within a supposedly unified and harmonious general psychiatric rational field (there are obvious conflicts between Goals X and Z, Y and D and E and B, for example)

health work is work to create autonomy by providing or maintaining foundations for achievement.

I have argued for this theory in several books, and do not reproduce this material here. However, a little knowledge of the foundations theory of health is necessary to understanding and using rational fields for total health promotion.

(The extract below is mostly adapted from Chapter 8 of *Practical Nursing Philosophy: The Universal Ethical Code*.[115])

THE BONES OF THE FOUNDATIONS THEORY OF HEALTH

The foundations theory of health has been in development for well over a decade, and forms a large part of three books.[60,98,128] Because it is explained more fully elsewhere, in what follows the discussion is restricted to a short general outline of the theory's basis, and a brief synopsis of its usefulness for health workers who wish to work for health with individuals and small groups.

The foundations theory of health is derived from conceptual analysis of the meaning of health (**Type 7** – see **Figure 2**), from study of other theories of health (**Type 7**), from empirical observation of work actually done in the name of health (**Type 1**), and from certain untestable beliefs about the morality of social arrangements (**Type 6**). My analysis of these matters has led me to conclude that any plausible account of health must understand the purpose of health work to be the identification, and if possible removal, of obstacles to worthwhile (or enhancing)[128] human potentials. That is:

> Work for health is essentially *enabling*. It is a question of providing the appropriate foundations to enable the achievement of personal and group potentials. Health in its different degrees is created by removing obstacles and by providing the basic means by which biological and chosen goals can be achieved.
>
> *A person's (optimum) state of health is equivalent to the state of the set of conditions which fulfil or enable a person to work to fulfil his or her realistic chosen and biological potentials. Some of these conditions are of the highest importance for all people. Others are variable dependent upon individual abilities and circumstances.*
>
> The actual degree of health that a person has at a particular time depends upon the degree to which these conditions are realised in practice.[128] (Quotation slightly changed from original.)

This idea can be depicted in the abstract (see **Figure 27**). The boxes in **Figure 27** may be described either as *conditions for* health or *constituents of* health (though ultimately only the latter understanding can be sustained[128]). Their importance, whichever way you look at them, is that they provide a platform for action. If a person can stand upon the four central blocks in good order then she will have a high level of health. If her boxes are in bad shape she will tend to have fewer options for fulfilling life performance than if they were sound.

How many different sorts of boxes there are, their exact content, and how important each is compared to the others is contestable, varies according to circumstance, and is

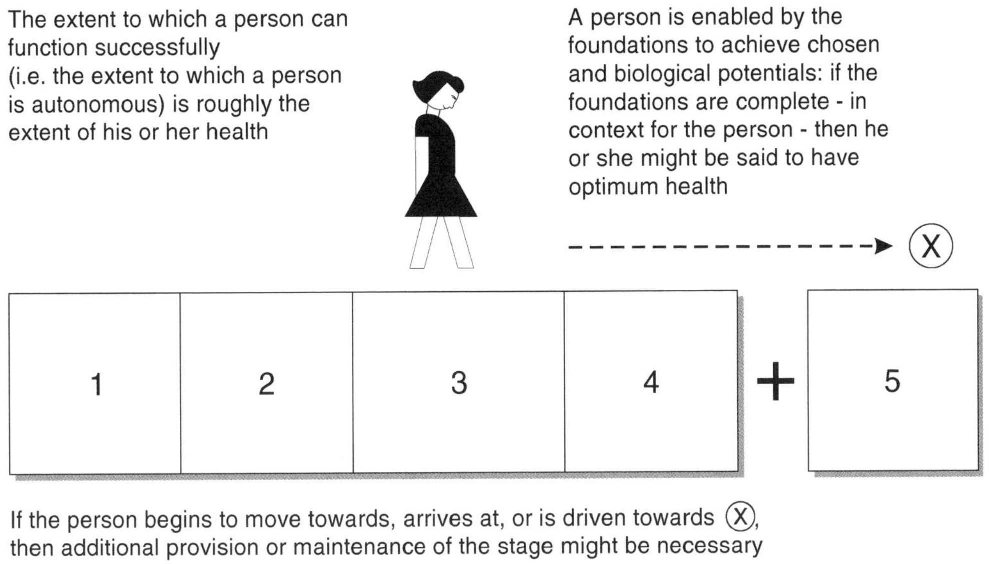
The extent to which a person can function successfully (i.e. the extent to which a person is autonomous) is roughly the extent of his or her health
A person is enabled by the foundations to achieve chosen and biological potentials: if the foundations are complete - in context for the person - then he or she might be said to have optimum health
X
1
2
3
4
+
5
If the person begins to move towards, arrives at, or is driven towards X, then additional provision or maintenance of the stage might be necessary

Figure 27 An abstract depiction of health. Reproduced with permission from *Practical Nursing Philosophy* by David Seedhouse ©2000, John Wiley & Sons Ltd, Chichester

at least partly a matter of human social judgement. On the foundations theory of health the numbered blocks shown in **Figure 27** have the following substance:

> Some of the foundations which make up health are of the highest importance for all people. These are:
>
> 1. The basic needs of food, drink, shelter, warmth and purpose in life.
> 2. Access to the widest possible information about all factors which have an influence on a person's life.
> 3. The skill and confidence to assimilate this information. In most societies literacy and numeracy are needed in older children and adults. People need to be able to understand how the information applies to them, and to be able to make reasoned decisions about what action to take in the light of their information.
> 4. The recognition that an individual is never totally isolated from other people and the external world. People are complex wholes who cannot be fully understood separated from the influence of their environment, which is itself a whole of which they are a part. People are not like marbles packed in boxes, where they are a community only because of their forced proximity. People are part of their whole surroundings, like cells in a single body. This fact compels the recognition that a person should not strive to fulfil personal potentials which will undermine the basic foundations for achievement of other people. In short, an essential condition for health in human beings who are aware of the implications of their actions is that they have an awareness of a basic duty they have because they are people in a community.
>
> Other foundations for achievement are bound to vary between individuals dependent upon which potentials can realistically be achieved. For instance, a diseased person, a person in a damp and dilapidated house, a person in prison, a fit young athlete, a terminal patient, and an expectant mother all need the central conditions which constitute part of their healths, but in addition they require other specific foundations in order to enable them to make the most of their present lives.[128]

The idea is that boxes 1–4 represent the central conditions for a fulfilling life, and that lack of (or serious defect in) them will severely impede a person in the achievement of enhancing potentials. Box 5 represents additional support made necessary by individual circumstance. When faced with a life crisis people sometimes find that the four central boxes, even in excellent condition, are of much less use than usual. If people are 'falling over the edge' of their platform they will need the support of a fifth box. That is, they will require the: '... other specific foundations [necessary] to enable them to make the most of their present lives...'[128]

The content of box 5 depends entirely upon the nature of the particular problem. Thus the fifth box may represent medical services and support; improved facilities for a disabled person; hospice care for a terminally ill man; special protection and counselling for a battered woman, and so on. The fifth box is needed when a particular life problem becomes bad enough to impede significantly a person's movement on the platform formed by the other four boxes. This box then either permanently extends the platform, substitutes for an irreparably damaged central box, or is the means by which a person is enabled to climb back onto her normal platform.

It will be immediately obvious that this notion of health does not have traditional medical provision as its focus. This is not a problem or an error, rather it is a logical consequence of the fact that work for health seeks to remove impediment to human achievement, and that problems that are tackled by medicine do not constitute a special category of impediment.[60] Just as a person becomes substantially immobilised in his life in general if he becomes seriously diseased or injured, so he is equally likely to be severely impeded in life if he does not have a home, or possesses no useful information, or has not been educated, or does not realise the extent to which he is formed by and depends on the existence of a community of others.

It may also appear that this theory of health implies that *any* effort to help people live better lives is work for health. However, while the theory certainly does extend the idea of health beyond medical endeavour, it nevertheless sets *limits* on the interests of health workers. The task for any genuine health worker working with an individual or a small group is to recognise the importance of the foundations in context – to identify with or for each individual those components which are lacking, or those which are most in need of renovation – and then to work on those aspects most appropriate to the skills of that health worker. In this way the theory begins to offer guidance to individual health workers, and may help establish practical priorities.

Crucially:

> ...work for health cannot be fully comprehensive – not all work should be thought to be health work. Such a state of affairs is not possible, nor is it desirable to have professional interference in the name of health covering all aspects of individual's lives. *Once suitable background conditions have been created, the achievement of the particular potentials that have been chosen is up to the individual and not the concern of health workers, although permanent maintenance work will often need to be carried out on the foundations.*
>
> The analogy of work for health is very close to the work needed to lay the foundations of a building. *Obstacles such as poor drainage, subsidence, awkward outcrops of rock (analogy: disease, illness, poor housing, unjustified discrimination, unemployment) have to be eliminated or overcome in some other way. Then firm foundations and reinforcements have to be added (analogy: good general education, confidence in thinking things through personally rather than relying on what one has been told, good opportunities for self-development). But, unlike the case of building*

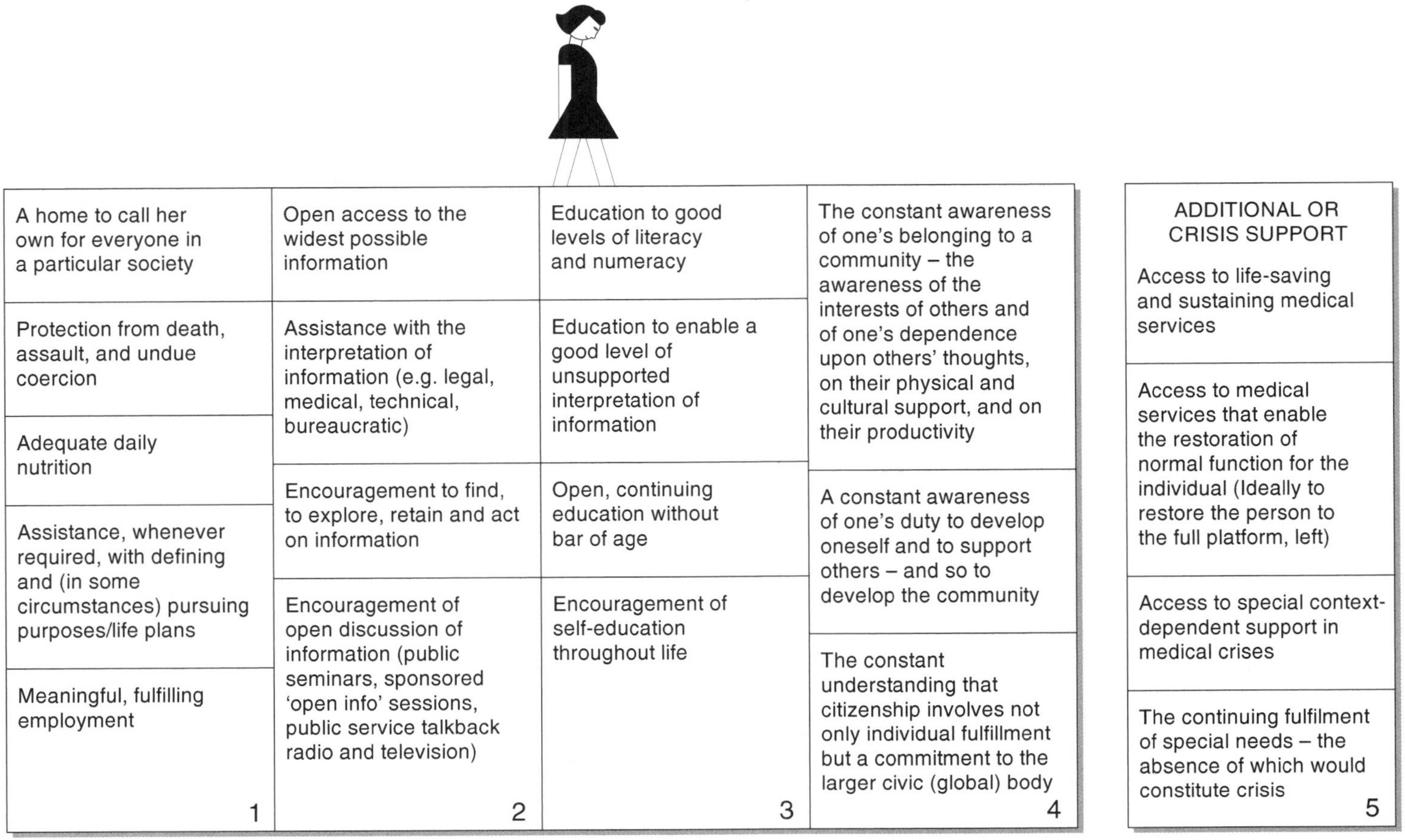
A home to call her own for everyone in a particular society
Protection from death, assault, and undue coercion
Adequate daily nutrition
Assistance, whenever required, with defining and (in some circumstances) pursuing purposes/life plans
Meaningful, fulfilling employment
1
Open access to the widest possible information
Assistance with the interpretation of information (e.g. legal, medical, technical, bureaucratic)
Encouragement to find, to explore, retain and act on information
Encouragement of open discussion of information (public seminars, sponsored 'open info' sessions, public service talkback radio and television)
2
Education to good levels of literacy and numeracy
Education to enable a good level of unsupported interpretation of information
Open, continuing education without bar of age
Encouragement of self-education throughout life
3
The constant awareness of one's belonging to a community – the awareness of the interests of others and of one's dependence upon others' thoughts, on their physical and cultural support, and on their productivity
A constant awareness of one's duty to develop oneself and to support others – and so to develop the community
The constant understanding that citizenship involves not only individual fulfillment but a commitment to the larger civic (global) body
4
ADDITIONAL OR CRISIS SUPPORT
Access to life-saving and sustaining medical services
Access to medical services that enable the restoration of normal function for the individual (Ideally to restore the person to the full platform, left)
Access to special context-dependent support in medical crises
The continuing fulfilment of special needs – the absence of which would constitute crisis
5

Figure 28 The foundations with more specific content. (Reproduced with permission from *Practical Nursing Philosophy* by David Seedhouse ©2000, John Wiley and Sons Ltd, Chichester)

> *construction, work for health should stop here.* What a person makes of the foundations he has is up to that person, as long as he possesses at least the essentials of the central conditions. Given this then an individual must be allowed to become the architect of her own destiny.[128] (Quotation slightly changed from the original.)

This understanding of health can be fleshed out (see **Figure 28** for example) though this is a general elucidation only. In fact in every case – whether the central figure is a person, group or still larger community – the specific content will vary dependent upon the figure's circumstances. One way to imagine this is to think of a one-armed bandit – or the departures board at a large airport. When the central figure changes so too does the content of the foundations – different concerns click into place dependent upon the prevailing situation and the aspirations of the central figure.

A family who have a badly handicapped neonate, a 40 year old with inoperable cancer and two young children, the increasingly forgetful septuagenarian – each will require the best foundations possible, but the exact nature, size and strength of each foundation will be different in each case. For example, the family with the handicapped neonate will require all five foundations in depth, and may particularly need boxes 4 and 5. In this case box 4 might be spelt out to mean all those supports already included in **Figure 28** plus extended contact with other families in similar situations. Box 5 will change from that shown in **Figure 28** and will reflect the specific needs of the baby (for medication, physiotherapy and so on) and the rest of the family (for counselling, grief support, extra financial support and so on).

MENTAL HEALTH PROMOTION SHOULD NOT BE A SEPARATE TASK ACCORDING TO THE FOUNDATIONS THEORY

Note that in keeping with the argument advanced in **Chapters Three** and **Four** of this book, the foundations theory makes no distinction between obstacles that are primarily tangible (lack of painkilling medicine, lack of money) and those that are primarily mental (the family's lack of understanding of their situation, a sense of loss, confusion about how to carry on). There is no need to divide these obstacles into separate categories for they are inextricably related: they are all part of the general problem. Attention to physical matters will have mental effects, and *vice versa*.

People are physical, thinking beings. Once we have no physical function we are dead. And if we cannot think, we might as well be dead.

While it sometimes makes sense to distinguish between physical and mental aspects of human life, it is neither conceptually nor practically desirable to distinguish between physical and mental health promotion. The fact that it is at times prudent to focus solely on, say, excessive grief or a physical addiction is a sign that single problems can sometimes be overwhelming – but it is not a proof that our mental and physical worlds are so different from one another that they require separate health promotion disciplines to cope with them. Consider how ridiculous it would be for a health promoter to focus exclusively on either the grief or the addiction. Grieving has physical consequences – loss of appetite, loss of motivation (a change in behaviour as well as a change in cognition), perhaps even loss of employment and friends. Physical addiction (if it even makes sense to talk of an addiction as exclusively physical) has mental effects – guilt, feelings of failure, disorientation as a result of the use of an addictive substance, and so on.

It is depressingly common to hear health professionals describe correlations between poverty and mental health problems when they take 'mental health problems' to mean only schizophrenia and the like. But of course poverty *itself* is a mental health problem (how many people are happy, fulfilled, creative and at ease in poverty?).

By using the understanding that health promotion means promoting autonomy (**Type 6** value: human autonomy is good and ought to be encouraged) it is possible to:

a. Incorporate parts of other rational fields (including psychiatry and mental health promotion) that may contribute to autonomy promotion.

b. Promote the health of individuals or groups by improving their foundations for achievement *and* their internal physical and mental capabilities without disconnecting them.

The foundational questions are always: how are these people impeded? and how best can we liberate their potentials? The answers may rest anywhere – in the individual, in relationships, in the social world, in the economy. The foundations theory of health sees people as integrated minds and bodies living with others in a complex and ever-changing environment.

c. Promote health without the need for absolute divisions within the health promotion rational field – and therefore without the need for a discipline called mental health promotion.

d. Re-orient psychiatry (were there to be the political will and ethical integrity to do this) in a way that creates a new, coherent and flexible rational field in which psychiatry can be practised in a way that is meaningfully and consistently devoted to the promotion of health.

How all this can actually be done is the subject of the final chapter.

CHA

Total Health Promotion

SUMMARY

This chapter:

- Explains that conventional health promotion is trapped within a rational field that exhibits almost all the errors of classification, value and logic explained in **Chapter Five**
- Makes the point that conventional health promotion does not recognise the importance of rational fields
- Shows how combining the rational field template with the foundations theory of health can render health promotion self-critical, comprehensive, ethically aware and explicitly focused
- Demonstrates how to display and compare basic rational fields in order to promote health, and provides several examples of how to undertake total health promotion using rational fields
- Provides a comprehensive list of the benefits of total health promotion, and urges its widespread adoption

◆

INTRODUCTION

This chapter explains how rational fields can be used to create autonomy – the ultimate goal of health promotion. If it is not already obvious why autonomy-creation is so important, here is a brief and upsetting account of misplaced and misunderstood 'work for health' – work for health in name only. This sort of thing happens with terrible monotony whenever practitioners are incapable of seeing over their high-walled rational fields:

> By mid-morning I was in custody, picked up by the police while standing in a bus garage, calling out about poisonous fumes in the earth. They locked me in a cell. I thought I was on the way down to Hades. Later they put me in a van and took me to a psychiatric hospital. I remember lying on the floor of a padded cell in my underclothes.
>
> The above scenario is a distillation of events from 18 years as a user of psychiatric services. Whatever else it may reveal, I believe it illustrates a major feature of life for those diagnosed as mentally ill: loss of control. Loss of control, whether truly lost or merely

> removed by others, and the attempt to re-establish that control have been central elements in my life since the age of 18. My argument is that the psychiatric system, as currently established, does too little to help people retain control of their lives through periods of emotional distress and does far too much to frustrate their subsequent efforts to regain self-control. Whatever power I now have over my life, I have, to a large extent, won in spite of rather than because of psychiatry...
>
> I find it significant that no psychiatric professional has ever advised me on how to cope with a breakdown beyond the blanket exhortation to keep on taking the drugs. My own experiences suggest that once I start to lose control again I am expected to admit powerlessness, hand myself over to the experts and count to 15,000...
>
> My argument against the psychiatric system is not that it is uncaring. I have met individuals at all levels – nurses, social workers, psychiatrists – who were clearly caring people and cared for me. By approaching my situation in terms of illness, by regarding me primarily as a recipient of care and treatment, the system has consistently underestimated my capacity to change and ignored the potential it may contain to assist that change.[128]

Total health promotion seeks to achieve exactly the opposite of loss of control, because this is the point of working for health.[127]

Chapter Six explains total health promotion, but it is far from the final word on the subject. Rather it is a sketchy blueprint – a selection of possibilities offered to health promoters seeking a more thoughtful, self-critical and ethically aware form of health promotion than the conformist version we have at present.

Total health promotion is an intellectually and socially challenging idea, and yet it is deeply practical as well. The total health promoter is free to question convention and to reject unsuitable health promotion purposes and methods. But at the same time she is at liberty to select the best aspects of conventional health promotion, if she believes they are the most effective and moral choice.

CONVENTIONAL HEALTH PROMOTION

Total health promotion is very different from the conventional version we have become used to over the past thirty years or so. The primary drive of total health promotion is to make both the source and internal workings of health-promoting rational fields completely explicit, whereas conventional health promoters are typically unaware of (or they deny) health promotion's beyond-the-evidence sources. Consequently it is most unusual to read about 'ethical issues' in health promotion – certainly such references are virtually unheard of in government and World Health Organisation (WHO) literature. The impression generally given is that conventional health promotion is obviously desirable: that health is the opposite of disease and illness, that disease and illness are obviously bad, and that therefore health promotion and all its methods are obviously good. Furthermore, since health promotion is obviously good it must be universally desirable, and therefore there can be no ethical issues in health promotion – or so the story goes.

Despite its demonstrable falsity, this simplistic view continues to dominate. An extensive explanation of its failings has been given in a companion volume,[63] so a full account is not given here. Suffice it to say that conventional health promotion is trapped in a rational field that exhibits at least seven **errors of classification, value and logic**.

Conventional Health Promotion's Errors of Classification, Value and Logic

Error 1. Using a single term to describe different states and processes (conventional health promotion uses 'health' to stand for all manner of states and processes)

Error 2. Acting as if a particular rational field is the only option, or acting as if only it is true and all others are false (conventional health promotion regards its declarations as commandments and its official bodies as oracles)

Error 3. Using different terms to describe states and processes that are fundamentally identical (conventional health promotion uses words like 'fitness', 'positive health', 'well-being' and – oblivious to grammatical error – even 'health prevention' to stand for anti-disease activities and outcomes)

Error 4. Knowingly constructing artificial divisions within or between rational fields (conventional health promotion constructs a massive divide between medically inspired health priorities (which is what conventional health promotion basically is) and non-medically inspired health priorities)

Error 5? Creating over-elaborate rational fields (conventional health promotion's fields are not particularly sophisticated – though they are very eclectic, so perhaps conventional health promotion is not guilty of this error)

Error 6. Not noticing or disregarding beyond-the-evidence assumptions and decisions (conventional health promotion is comprehensively guilty of this – for example, conventional health promotion rarely if ever seriously debates the morality of its projects, and yet it takes only a moment's thought to see that campaigns for mass immunisation, the obligatory consumption of fluoridated water, and advertising drives to frighten young people away from illicit drug use are morally controversial)

Error 7. Failing to provide comprehensive explanations and justifications of the value-judgements and instincts that make up the perimeter of the field (conventional health promotion is comprehensively guilty of this too – to persuade a parent to take a risk by immunising her child in the interest of other children quite obviously requires a value-judgement, and the decision not to explain this value-judgement to those on the receiving end of it requires a detailed moral defence, at the very least)

Error 8. Perpetuating rational fields that incorporate contradictory notions (conventional health promotion's appearance of 'obviousness' obscures significant clashes of purpose and morality)[63]

Vaguely expressed, conventional health promotion's rational field looks roughly like **Figure 29**.

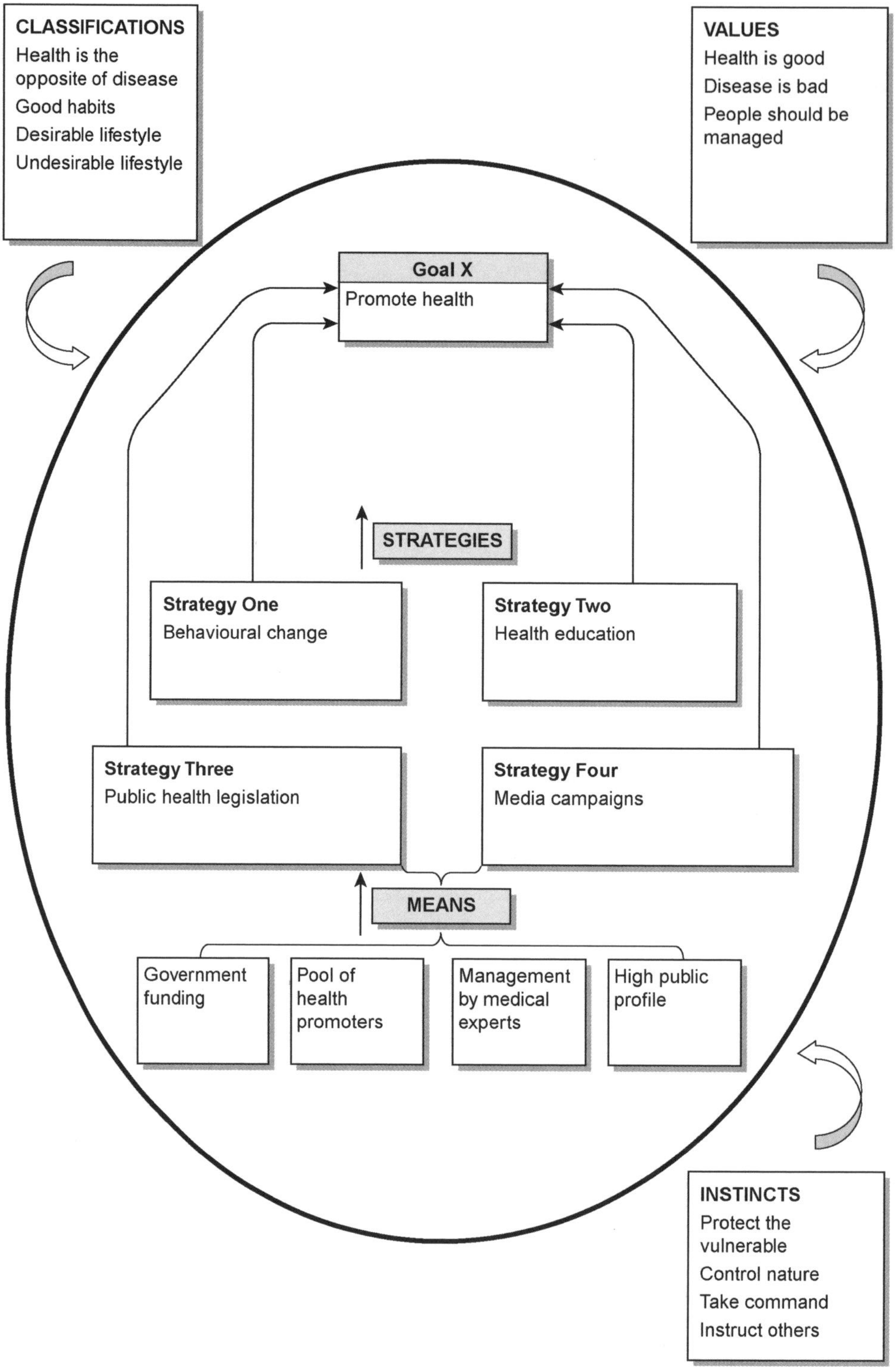

Figure 29 Conventional health promotion's rational field (vaguely and generally expressed)

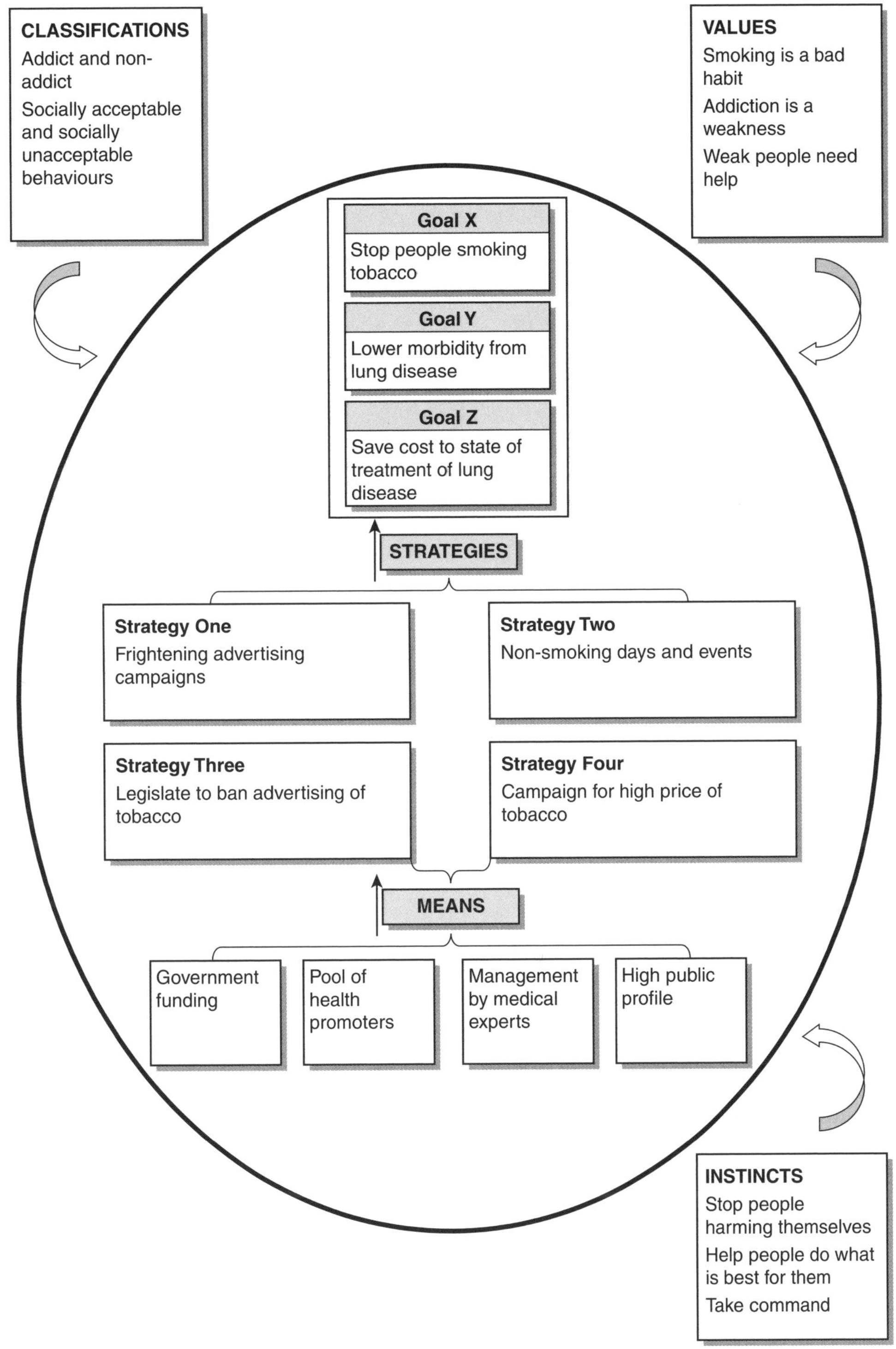

Figure 30 A typical specific conventional health promotion rational field

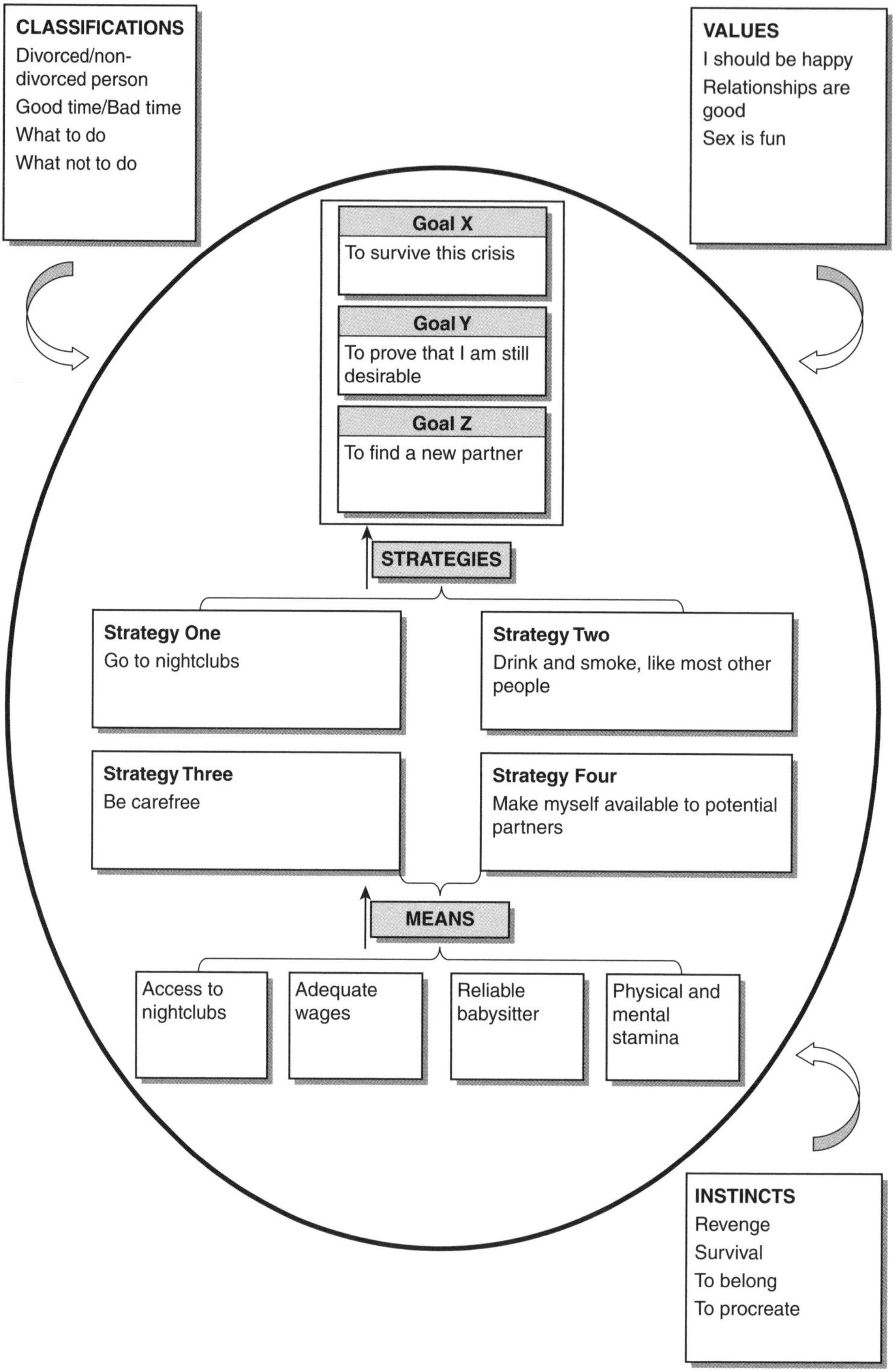

Figure 31 A recently divorced 35-year-old woman's 'social life' rational field

A typical more specific conventional health promotion rational field is depicted in **Figure 30**.

These fields look very straightforward when they are seen in isolation – indeed, reading them one can almost understand why so many health promoters cannot comprehend how there is anything to object to in conventional health promotion. However, set **Figure 30** next to **Figure 31**, and things instantly become less assured.

To the recently divorced 35 year old, smoking is not a bad thing, indeed she needs to smoke because it reminds her of the days before her recently and utterly failed marriage. What's more, she desperately wants to be part of the crowd, and most of the crowd smoke. Health promotion advice to quit smoking falls on her deaf ears, and yet conventional health promotion tactics may affect her nevertheless. If, for example, the conventional health promotion lobby succeeds in raising the price of cigarettes, this might have adverse consequences for the youngish divorcee – if the price goes up a lot she may not be able to afford to go out as much and may therefore be less able to reach her immediate life goals. And she may be made to feel bad or guilty about smoking, when additional guilt and recrimination is one of the last things she needs just now.

If you ignore all the rational fields that surround the conventional health promotion field then conventional health promotion can seem blessedly unproblematic. However, once you acknowledge the surrounding fields, the health promotion task changes completely. For example, the total health promoter, if faced with the divorcee, would be primarily concerned to raise her autonomy. With this in mind he would be quite uninterested in her short-term smoking. He would, however, be concerned to help her clarify her goals – are they compatible? Is looking for a new partner in night clubs the best way to weather the crisis? Is proving her desirability the best way to find the most suitable partner? The total health promoter would be particularly interested in her platform of means, with a view to bolstering it according to the foundations understanding of health, if possible.

THE TOTAL HEALTH PROMOTER MUST ALWAYS TAKE A BROAD VIEW OF PREVAILING RATIONAL FIELDS

The world is made up of an unfathomably complex set of purposes. Therefore, whenever the total health promoter wants to promote health she must distinguish salient sets of rational fields from the great ocean of rational fields in which we all swim. This is indeed a challenge, but it is not an impossible one. We distinguish salient rational fields all the time in life in general, though we are rarely aware of it (we do it as we decide which house to purchase, decide whether to resign a post, decide whether to punish our children, decide on a partner and so on).

AN ILLUSTRATIVE EXAMPLE OF HOW TO SET RATIONAL FIELDS OUT SIDE BY SIDE

To understand the basic idea, consider this example. Cancer cells are rational fields, and a person is a rational field. These rational fields are usually incompatible – indeed

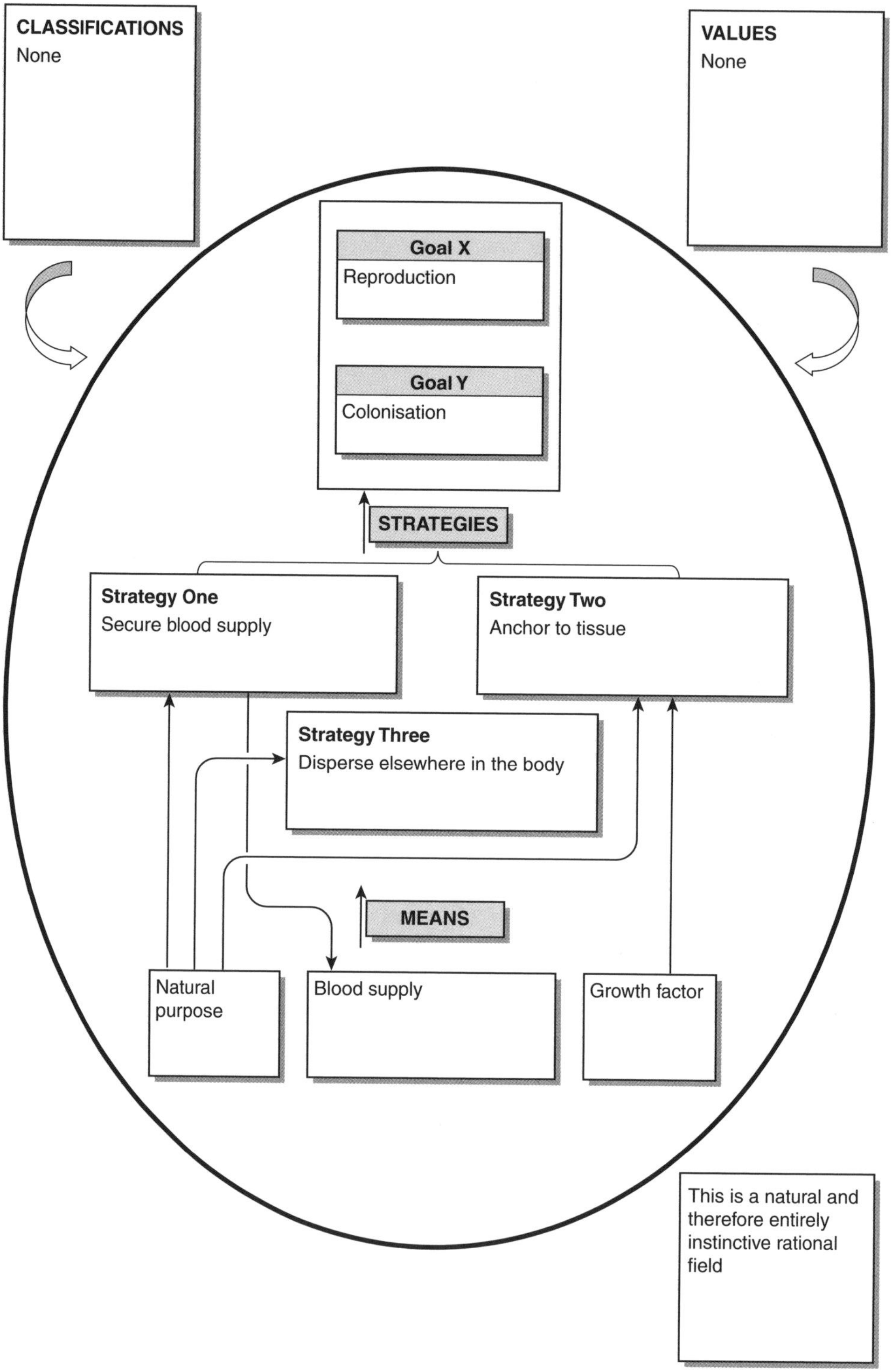

Figure 32 Rational field C

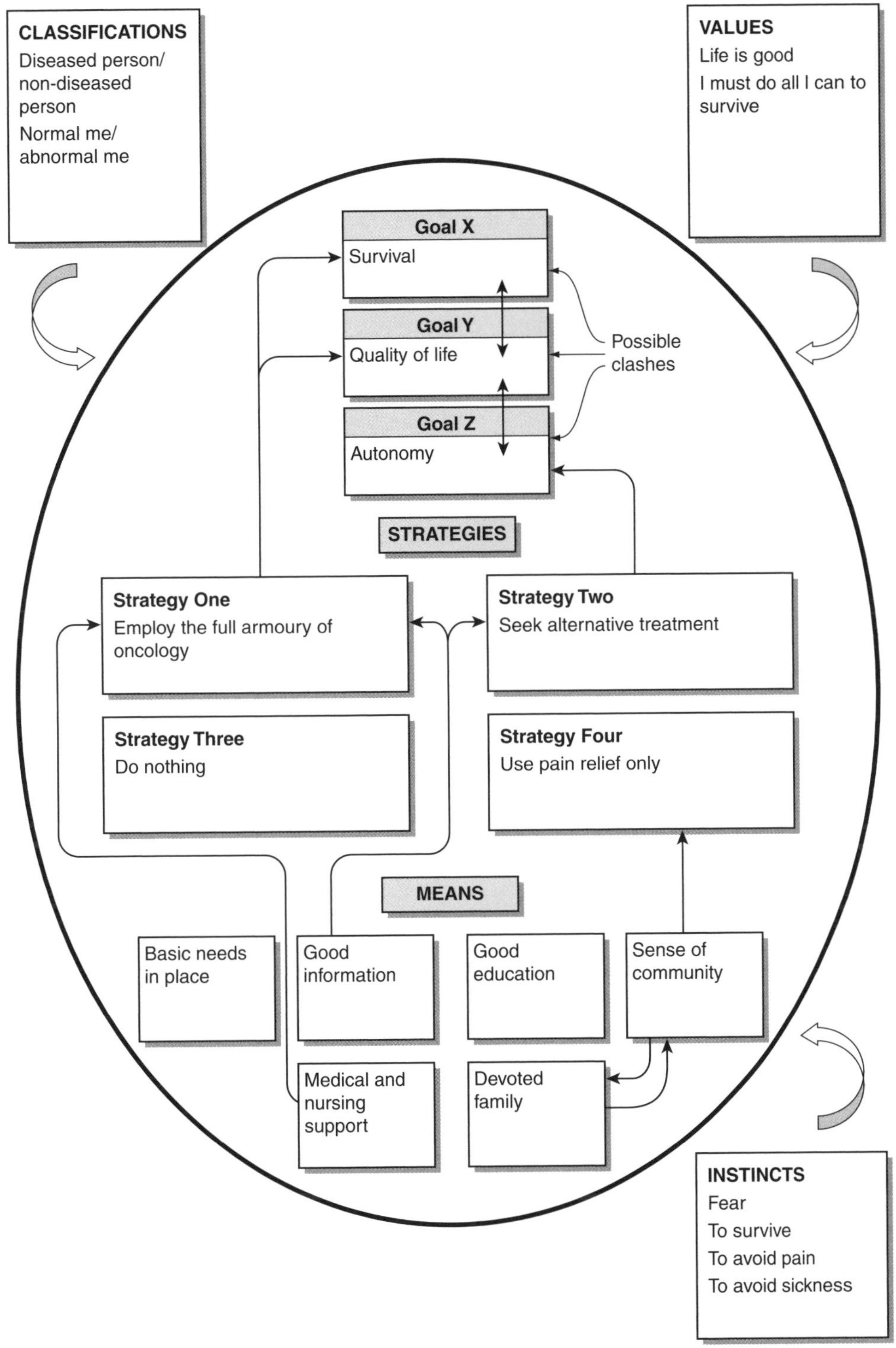

Figure 33 Rational Field P (arrows illustrative only)

they are mostly mutually destructive. Display them using the rational field template and their rationality is obvious. Moreover, casting them as rational fields makes the various responses to them crystal clear (and this is true of displaying rational fields in general – so much that is usually hidden instantly becomes visible).

Call the cancer cells Rational Field C and the person Rational Field P. Now take the roughly completed rational field templates in **Figures 32** and **33**.

Just by focusing on the two rational fields, we have at least three health promotion options:

1. Try to change Rational Field C
2. Try to change or develop Rational Field P – decide on a key goal and strategy and ensure the fullest possible means are in place
3. Try to render Rational Fields C and P compatible within a larger rational field

Deciding on options after reviewing relevant rational fields is an important part of the total health promotion challenge. In this case, as always, the decision to prefer option 1, 2 or 3 will draw on both evidence and non-evidence.

Scientists trying to find ways of defeating cancer naturally enough go for option 1. As they do so scientists aim either to change the goals of the cancer cells, or to make the cells stop reproducing,[129] or to affect the cells' strategies (for example, to prevent the cells securing a blood supply[130]) or to affect the means (for example to eliminate growth factors[131]).

Health workers trying to help patients deal with having cancerous cells also work on rational fields. They usually begin by helping the sufferer define her main goals and if necessary rank them in order of priority (for example, survival and quality of life may no longer be compatible because of cancer therapy, at least in the short term). After that – if possible – they try to provide the most potentially autonomy-promoting means, and try to link means to goals by means of the most appropriate strategy.

A further alternative is to try to unite the two rational fields in some way – to make them compatible. For example, it may be possible to absorb Rational Fields C and P within a further rational field – perhaps to do with 'religious experience' or 'spiritual awareness' or 'meaning of life' – the existence of which means that Fields C and P could be seen as harmonious (the cancer sufferer might become reconciled to her mortality and significantly increase her quality of life as a result).

THE TROUBLED ADOLESCENT – A FULLY WORKED EXAMPLE OF HOW TO CARRY OUT TOTAL HEALTH PROMOTION

Recall Peter Breggin's alternative view of 'adolescent schizophrenia':

> People are often labelled schizophrenic during their teen years. Adolescence, with its struggle to form identity in the face of unleashed passions, easily gets called 'mental

illness'. Whether adolescents become labelled mentally ill often depends mostly on the love, patience and tolerance of the adults who surround them.[35]

The common situation of the lost adolescent – the mixed-up kid – is interpreted in all manner of ways. As a rule, each interpreter believes his interpretation is correct. However, put different interpretations together as competing rational fields, and such confidence must surely be shaken (see **Figures 34–37**).

These are very simplified depictions of a fairly common adolescent situation. Of course they do not tell the full story. What's more the values and instincts depicted are sparse. Reality is much more complicated than this. However, there are certainly some values and instincts behind each of these rational fields, since rational fields cannot exist without them. So, if the illustrated speculations are inadequate, the question is: what actual values and instincts are in play?

These simple illustrations contain – at least in my view – a grain of truth and indicate a solid way forward for the health promoter in this case. Crucially, the total health promoter should not prejudge the matter as a 'psychiatric problem', a 'social problem' or an 'adolescents' problem' – or any other preordained sort of problem – the total health promoter must try to assess the situation by setting out the salient rational fields as clearly and fully as possible, comparing and assessing them, and then trying to work out what creating autonomy means, and after that working out how actually to bring it about.

WHAT THE TOTAL HEALTH PROMOTER CAN DO FOR THE TROUBLED ADOLESCENT

Remember that the perimeters or walls of rational fields are composed of classifications, values and **just is** instincts. Given this, using the rational field template, the total health promoter is systematically able to do three very important things:

STEP 1: She can analyse each rational field independently, by asking **ten clarifying questions**

STEP 2: She can compare and contrast various salient (often competing) rational fields, again by asking **ten clarifying questions**

STEP 3: She can supply the bones of the foundations theory of health in order to devise the most health-promoting rational field

Here's how these three steps might work out in the case of the troubled adolescent, Matthew Parrish.

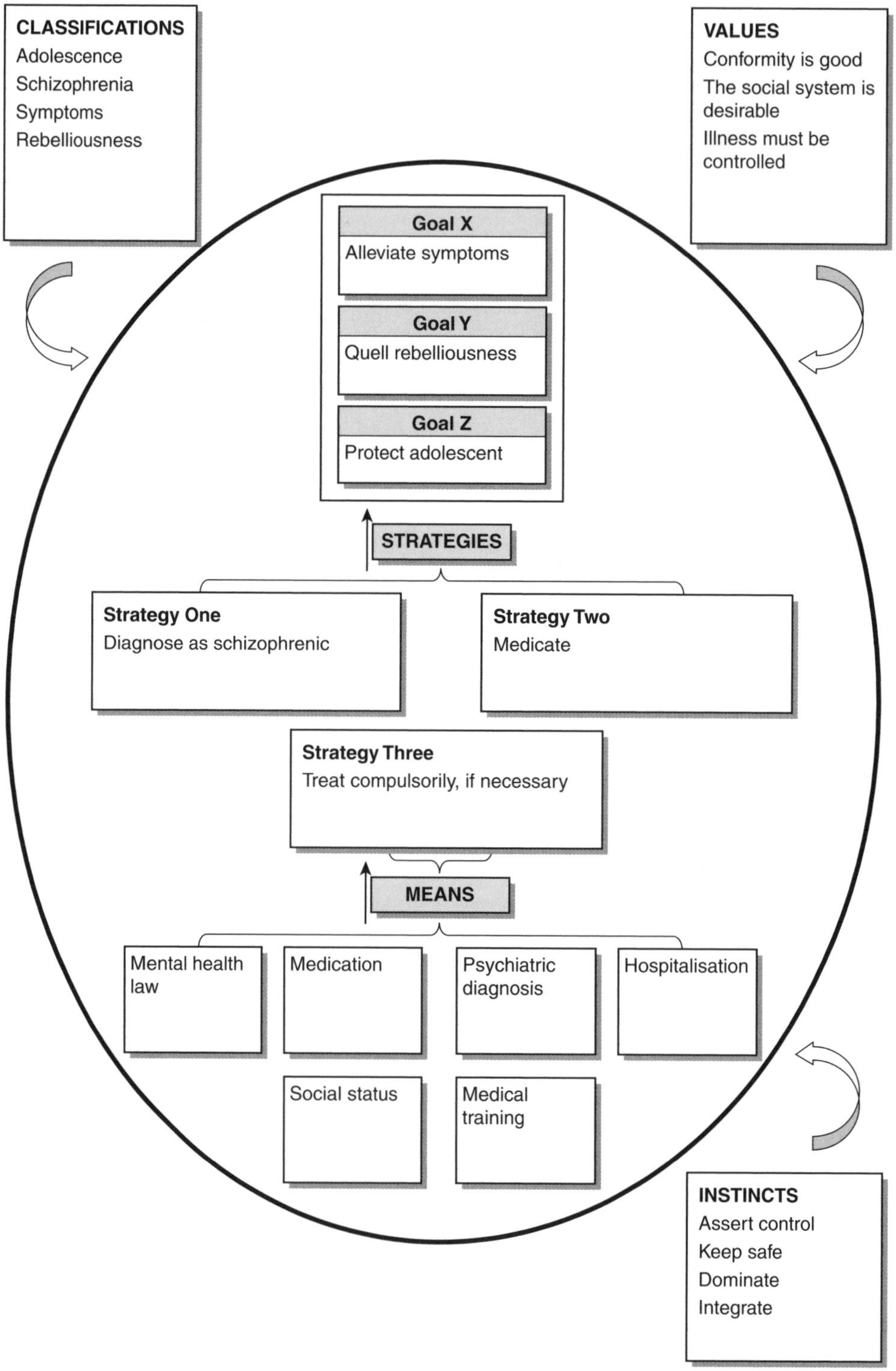

Figure 34 The psychiatric view of the troubled adolescent (illustrative)

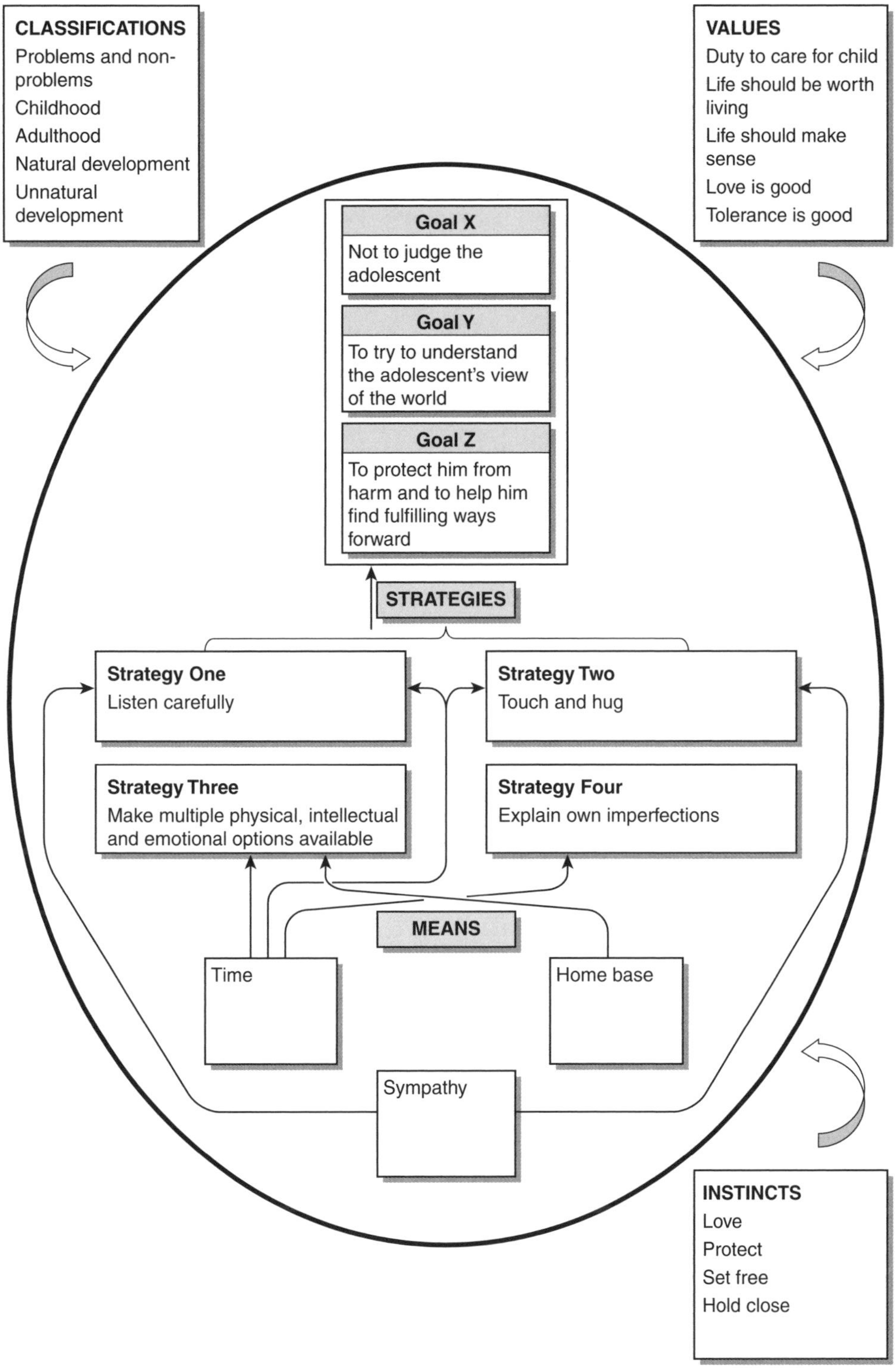

Figure 35 The supportive parent's view of what he can do for the troubled adolescent (illustrative)

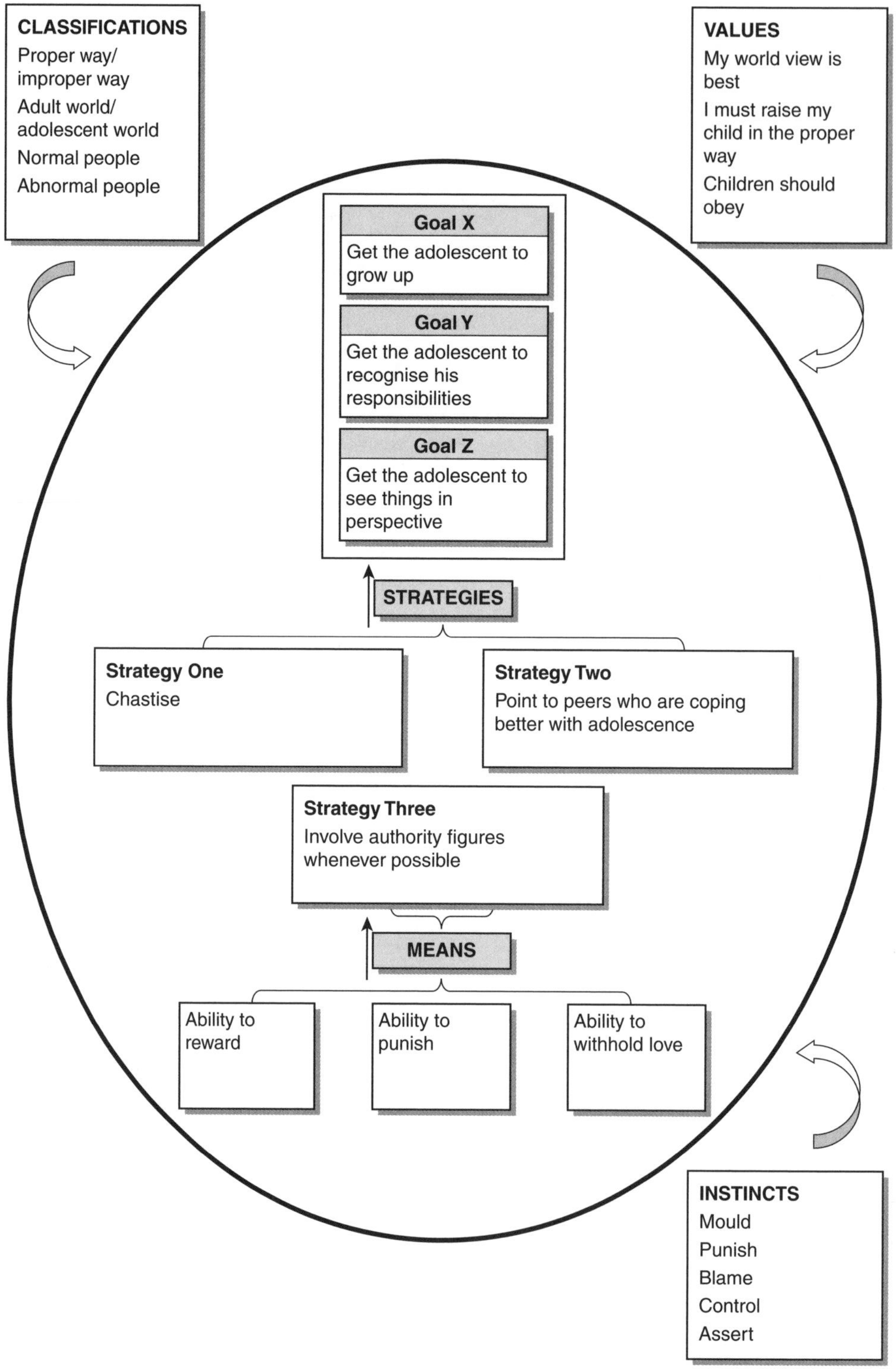

Figure 36 The unsupportive parent's view

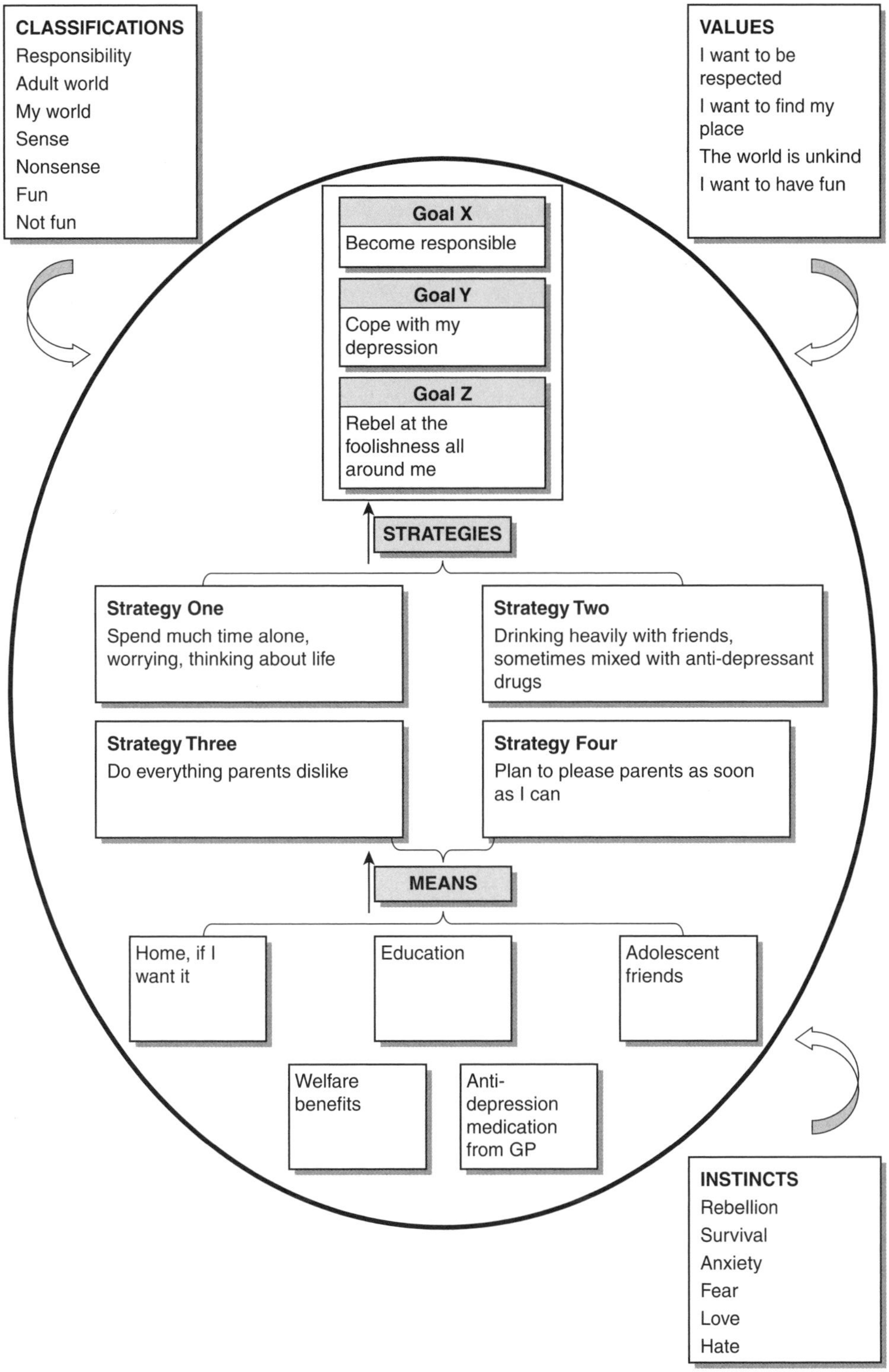

Figure 37 The adolescent's natural field (illustrative)

STEP 1: Analyse Each Rational Field

Rational fields may be analysed by asking **ten clarifying questions**.

TEN CLARIFYING QUESTIONS

1. ARE THE RATIONAL FIELD'S GOALS COMPATIBLE?
2. IF NO, IS IT POSSIBLE TO SELECT COMPATIBLE GOALS ONLY, OR TO CHANGE THE GOALS?
3. ARE THE GOALS REALISTIC GIVEN PRIMARY SURROUNDING RATIONAL FIELDS?
4. DO THE GOALS CREATE THE MOST AUTONOMY IN THE SUBJECT(S) WHO INHABIT OR WILL INHABIT THE FIELD?
5. ARE THE GOALS DESIRED BY THE SUBJECT(S) WHO INHABIT OR WILL INHABIT THE FIELD?
6. ARE THE STRATEGIES/MEANS APPROPRIATE TO THE ACHIEVEMENT OF THE GOALS?
7. IF NO, WHAT POSITIVE GOALS CAN BE ACHIEVED USING THESE STRATEGIES/MEANS IN CONTEXT?
8. WHAT BEYOND-THE-EVIDENCE ASSUMPTIONS HAVE CREATED THE RATIONAL FIELD?
9. IS THE FIELD RIGID, FLEXIBLE OR DISINTEGRATING?
10. IS IT POSSIBLE TO ALTER THE DEGREE OF RIGIDITY OF THE FIELD?

REMEMBER THAT THE PURPOSE OF TOTAL HEALTH PROMOTION IS TO WORK OUT HOW TO DESIGN REALISTIC RATIONAL FIELDS, ABLE TO CREATE THE BROADEST AUTONOMY.

For this book's purposes it is not necessary to offer a comprehensive analysis of the situation (in any case, little circumstantial detail has been given). However, in order to show the general shape of total health promotion strategy, this is how the psychiatry rational field and the adolescent's rational field stand up to scrutiny.

The Psychiatric Rational Field (Figure 34) Analysed Using the Ten Clarifying Questions

1. ARE THE GOALS COMPATIBLE?

Goal X (alleviate symptoms) and **Goal Y** (quell rebelliousness) are compatible – anti-psychotic medication can achieve both. However, whether these goals are compatible with **Goal Z** is a different matter, and depends on what is meant by 'protect'.

The key terms in rational fields are often loosely defined by the walls – by instincts, values and classifications. Seen from this particular psychiatric view of the world, 'protect' means calm Matthew down and keep him safe until he is ready to accept that the adult world is a desirable place, and that he has a role to play in its future.

2. IF NO, IS IT POSSIBLE TO SELECT COMPATIBLE GOALS ONLY, OR TO CHANGE THE GOALS?

For the psychiatric field, assuming that the aim is to render the field as rational as possible, the psychiatrist's task must be to make the nature of 'protect' clear, and to ensure that the field's means, strategies and goals are consistent.

3. ARE THE GOALS REALISTIC GIVEN PRIMARY SURROUNDING RATIONAL FIELDS?

Yes, given that psychiatry's rational field is socially sanctioned and that the medication can achieve the field's goals.

4. DO THE GOALS CREATE THE MOST AUTONOMY IN THE SUBJECT(S) WHO INHABIT OR WILL INHABIT THE FIELD?

This is highly arguable, since the point of this psychiatric rational field is to stop the adolescent doing what he wants, on the ground that it is not in his best interest. Even if you agree entirely with the psychiatric rational field you must accept that the autonomy question is controversial, not least since the psychiatric therapy deliberately seeks to limit autonomy (albeit with the intention of increasing it in the long run).

5. ARE THE GOALS DESIRED BY THE SUBJECT(S) WHO INHABIT OR WILL INHABIT THE FIELD?

To answer this question we must inspect the adolescent's rational field, since Matthew is the target of the health promotion intervention.

6. ARE THE STRATEGIES/MEANS APPROPRIATE TO THE ACHIEVEMENT OF THE GOALS?

Yes, they work.

7. IF NO, WHAT POSITIVE GOALS CAN BE ACHIEVED USING THESE STRATEGIES/MEANS IN CONTEXT?

N/A

8. WHAT BEYOND-THE-EVIDENCE ASSUMPTIONS HAVE CREATED THE RATIONAL FIELD?

See the classifications, values and instincts expressed in **Figure 34**.

9. IS THE FIELD RIGID, FLEXIBLE OR DISINTEGRATING?

To answer this the health promoter has to check for the **eight errors of classification, value and logic** listed in **Chapter Five**, of which the following are relevant in this case:

Error 2. Acting as if a particular rational field is the only option, or acting as if only it is true and all others are false

Error 6. Not noticing or disregarding beyond-the-evidence decisions and assumptions

Error 7. Failing to provide comprehensive explanations and justifications of the value-judgements and instincts that make up the perimeter of the field

Conclusion: the present rational field is rigid.

10. IS IT POSSIBLE TO ALTER THE DEGREE OF RIGIDITY OF THE FIELD?

Yes, but to do so one would need to incorporate additional goals drawn from one or more of the other rational fields.

The Adolescent's Rational Field (Figure 37) Analysed

1. ARE THE GOALS COMPATIBLE?

No, they are not.

2. IF NO, IS IT POSSIBLE TO SELECT COMPATIBLE GOALS ONLY, OR TO CHANGE THE GOALS?

When working directly with the subject(s) of the intervention this is not for the total health promoter to decide alone. The total health promoter must work with the person in question and must – of course – have a background theory of health to help her propose the best ways forward for the troubled adolescent, and to set limits in her intervention.

3. ARE THE GOALS REALISTIC GIVEN PRIMARY SURROUNDING RATIONAL FIELDS?

Not particularly. Most salient rational fields seem to be predominantly hostile to Matthew's rather confused intentions.

4. DO THE GOALS CREATE THE MOST AUTONOMY IN THE SUBJECT(S) WHO INHABIT OR WILL INHABIT THE FIELD?

No, because they are inconsistent and out of step with what is going on around Matthew.

5. ARE THE GOALS DESIRED BY THE SUBJECT(S) WHO INHABIT OR WILL INHABIT THE FIELD?

Apparently.

6. ARE THE STRATEGIES/MEANS APPROPRIATE TO THE ACHIEVEMENT OF THE GOALS?

Strategies 1–3 seem most compatible with **Goal Z** ('rebel at the foolishness around me'). Strategy 4 seems consistent with **Goal X**, if pleasing one's parents really is the same as becoming responsible, that is.

7. IF NO, WHAT POSITIVE GOALS CAN BE ACHIEVED USING THESE STRATEGIES/MEANS IN CONTEXT?

Again, this question is best addressed once the total health promoter is armed with a purposive theory of health. Or, to put it another way, once she has created – or has suggested – an optimally health-promoting rational field.

8. WHAT BEYOND-THE-EVIDENCE ASSUMPTIONS HAVE CREATED THE RATIONAL FIELD?

See the classifications, values and instincts expressed in **Figure 37** – of course, there are almost certainly many more beyond-the-evidence assumptions driving the adolescent, and specialist attention of some kind may be necessary to reveal them.

9. IS THE FIELD RIGID, FLEXIBLE OR DISINTEGRATING?

It is very obviously disintegrating.

10. IS IT POSSIBLE TO ALTER THE DEGREE OF RIGIDITY OF THE FIELD?

Yes, the field can be made more stable by addressing inconsistencies between goals, re-examining strategies and means, exposing the beyond-the-evidence assumptions (which may be hidden both from Matthew and from the other people involved), and devising ways to find a better fit between the adolescent's primary rational field and the closest surrounding rational fields.

STEP 2: Compare and Contrast Salient Rational Fields

To tackle **STEP 2** the total health promoter must display the most relevant rational fields. In this case, she should lay out **Figures 33** to **37**, placing them side by side.

It goes without saying that by doing this – and by filling in any simple rational field template at all – the total health promoter cannot claim to have grasped the whole truth of the situation. If there is such a thing as the absolute truth about the human experience, it is far too complicated for us poor humans to grasp. For example, even in this small case of adolescent turmoil, four different human experiences are pulled together – how can anyone properly understand every one of these and their interactions?

Furthermore, the creation of rational fields – and also the comparison of rational fields – involves both evidence and non-evidence. And in the world of health promotion there is always a significant proportion of beyond-the-evidence input – the health promoter has values herself, she classifies things in particular ways, and she has biological instincts too. All this means that like everything else from beyond-the-evidence, the health promoter's interpretation of the situation and the rational fields involved is a *speculation*. It isn't science – though it can make use of science – and it isn't certain. And given this, it is of the greatest importance that the source of this speculation is open and clear to everyone (and this is why the total health promoter is honest – she admits both her essential prejudices and her uncertainties, and she also says 'if you want me to help you then you ought to know about the theory of health that I am committed to').

How do the four rational fields compare in this case? Again, analysis may be initiated by means of the **ten clarifying questions**:

1. ARE THE RATIONAL FIELDS' GOALS COMPATIBLE?

No, they are not. The most obvious conflicts (to me) are:

a. Psychiatric **Goal Y** (quell rebelliousness) and the adolescent's **Goal Z** (rebel at the foolishness all around me)
b. Psychiatric **Goal Z** (protect adolescent) and the adolescent's **Goal X** (become responsible) – how will Matthew learn to become responsible if all responsibility is taken away from him?
c. Supportive parent's **Goal X** (not to judge the adolescent) and unsupportive parent's **Goal X** (get the adolescent to grow up)

There are other conflicts, of course, some of which the health promoter should note and investigate further. There are also some compatible goals – for example, psychiatric **Goal X** (alleviate symptoms) and the adolescent's **Goal Y** (cope with my depression), and these too could be investigated further (would medication help, or should it be a last resort?).

2. IF NO, SELECT COMPATIBLE GOALS ONLY, OR CHANGE GOALS

This is a hard call, but it needs to be made. It can be done, but only once the foundations theory of health has been fed into the rational field template.

3. ARE THE GOALS REALISTIC GIVEN PRIMARY SURROUNDING RATIONAL FIELDS?

The goals tend to compete with each other. When compared to further surrounding rational fields the picture only becomes more complicated. The adolescent's friends want different things for Matthew, his school wishes to wash its hands of him, and on top of this the 'let's get a job' rational field is becoming harder and harder for the adolescent to inhabit.

All this is obvious enough without rational field templates, of course.

4. DO THE GOALS CREATE THE MOST AUTONOMY IN THE SUBJECT(S) WHO INHABIT OR WILL INHABIT THE FIELD?

This is another tricky question. Each protagonist – apart perhaps from Matthew, who may find it hard to see the relevance of the question – will defend their manufactured rational field in this regard. Even the psychiatrist, whose regime will decrease the boy's autonomy in the short term, is bound to claim that the therapy will bring about the most autonomy in the long run.

Once again, to answer this question we need a proper theory of health, and we need to assess the evidence, if we can (what usually happens to psychiatrically treated adolescents, for example?).

5. ARE THE GOALS DESIRED BY THE SUBJECT(S) WHO INHABIT OR WILL INHABIT THE FIELD?

This is a crucial question – what does the adolescent want? Which is the best rational field for Matthew? Can he accept an autonomy-creating compromise?

The remainder of the clarifying questions add little in this case. Thus the total health promoter should go to **STEP 3**, in order to work out how to design realistic rational fields able to create the greatest autonomy.

STEP 3: Feed the Foundations Theory into the Rational Field

As we have seen at **STEP 2**, use of the rational field template begins to fall flat in the absence of a substantial understanding of the point of health work. Without a clearly purposive standpoint it is difficult, if not impossible, to arbitrate between the various rational fields in play.

This problem can be solved by means of the foundations theory.

The foundations theory of health was briefly summarised in **Chapter Five**. Its basic inspiration is that work for health is work to remove obstacles to fulfilling biological and chosen human potentials – to create autonomy, in other words. It may be that some health work – for example, giving medication which has side-effects – diminishes autonomy in the short term. However, this and other diminishments *may* be acceptable so long as the intention is to create autonomy for the subject or subjects of the health work, as quickly and effectively as possible.

The foundations theory has other features – for example, it is designed so that the more autonomy the subject has the less right the health worker has to continue to intervene. These features are fully explained elsewhere,[127] and they ought to be thoroughly understood by anyone who seriously wishes to undertake total health promotion. However, for present purposes, it is enough to show how the foundations theory and the rational field template can constructively combine (the method described below can be used in any health promotion task).

The primary focus of the foundations theory of health is on the *means for health* – specifically on the 5+ boxes that form the foundations and are illustrated in **Figures 27** and **28** in this book. The idea is that if these boxes are generally sound then any person or group (depicted by the central figure) will have good health, even if he, she or they have a disease or illness. Given decent foundations they should be in a good position to formulate their life goals, which are not usually the concern of the health promoter.

Total health promotion changes the balance of the foundations theory a little, since it is based on assessing rational fields, which are essentially composed of means, strategy *and* goals. This is not a bad thing, since it enables the health promoter to help the subject(s) by using logical analysis, and by helping them explicitly compare their situation with the surrounding situation, using rational field templates. The health promoter must still be aware that her task is to liberate the person or persons to pursue the goals they want to pursue by providing the best possible foundations – but this can be even better facilitated by using the rational field.

How can it be done?

First, take the **general foundations rational field template** shown in **Figure 38**.

Leave the goals and strategies blank. Now, working always with the subject of the intervention – in this case the adolescent – take the other existing rational fields you

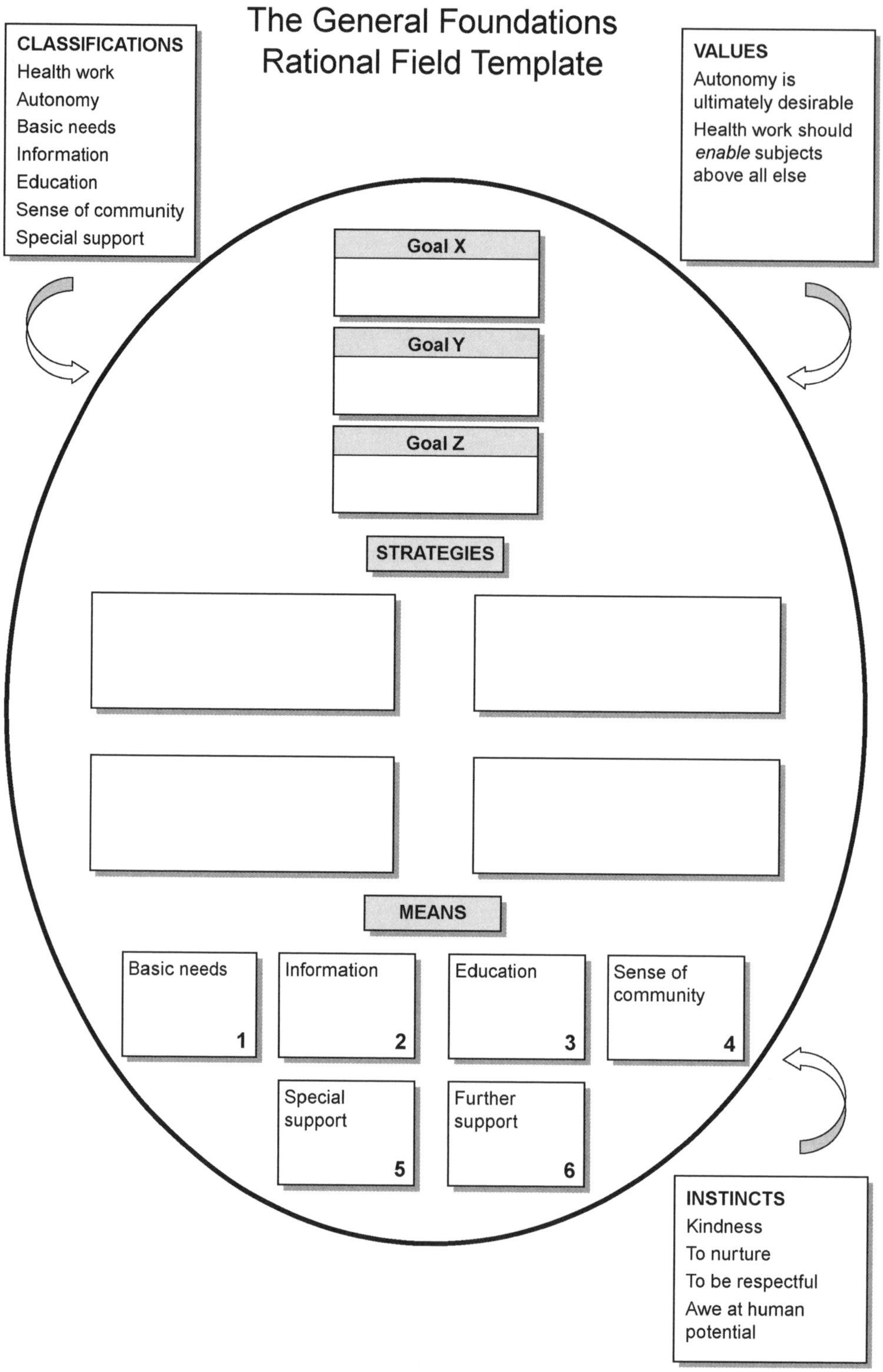

Figure 38 The General Foundations Rational Field Template

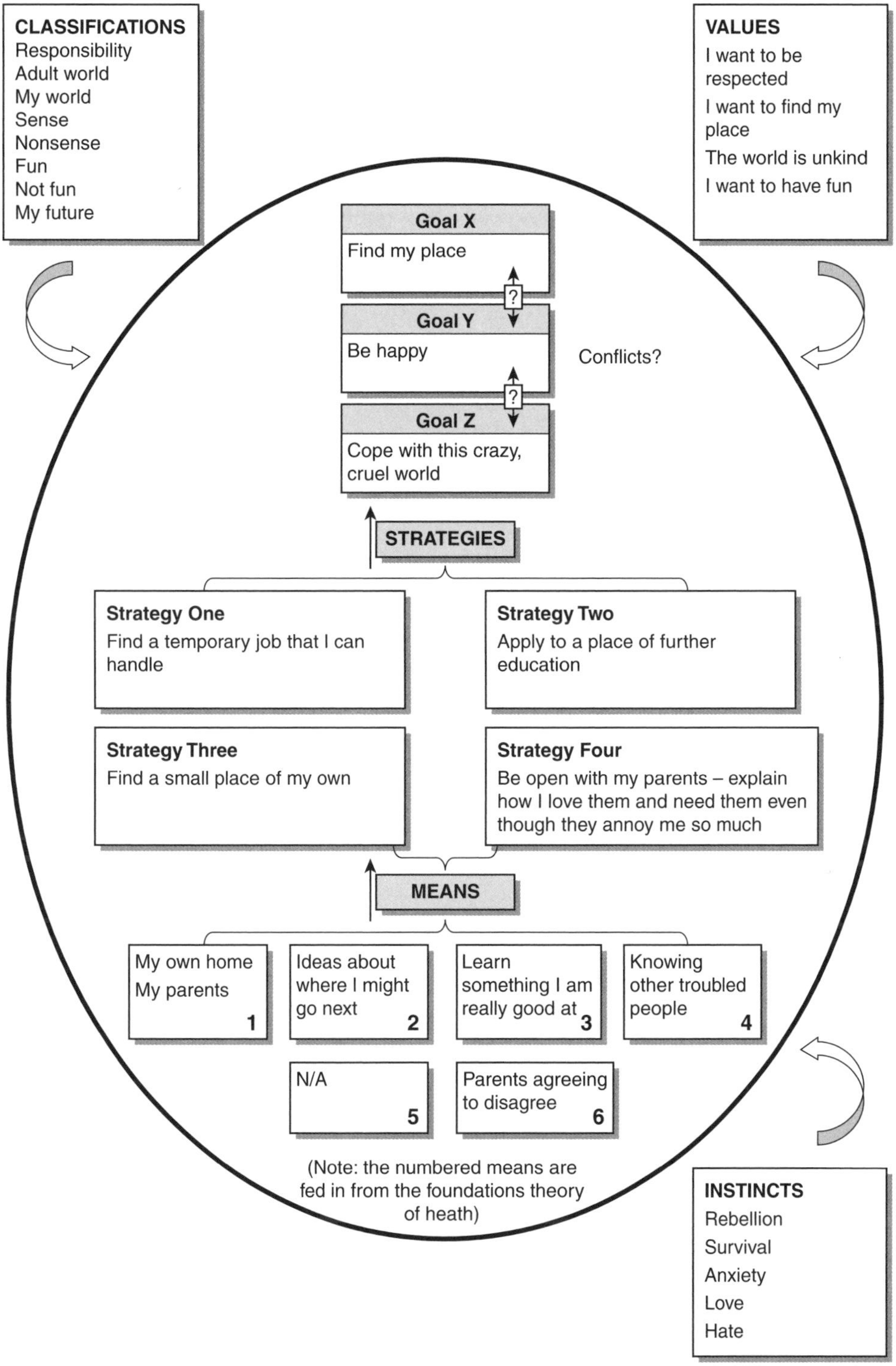

Figure 39 A possible foundational rational field manufactured to maximise the autonomy of the troubled adolescent

have identified, including the adolescent's own. (In other words, display **Figures 34–37** *for the adolescent to inspect.*)

Second, discuss these fields frankly with the adolescent, pointing out goals and consequences, logic and illogic, good strategies for achieving the goals and not so good strategies. Then begin to have the adolescent rethink his goals – what does he really want to do now, and what might he be doing in, say, a year or so? Is it possible to draw up a set of goals more in keeping with what he really wants; goals that are a better fit with the present surrounding rational fields?

Third, after a while, and in order to help with this process, suggest using the **general foundations rational field template**, of course with the values, instincts and classifications as fully expressed as possible (these should be more extensive than illustrated – like all the rational field figures in this book, **Figure 38** is illustrative only). Ask the adolescent to interpret the means (boxes 1–6) for his own context. What are his needs? Are they met? What information does he have? What more does he need?

Continue this process, tentatively detailing means, goals and eventually strategies: given these means and these goals how best can you go about using the means to achieve your goals? Leave it open to you and the adolescent to choose from any of the other templates already completed, and also to add in new ideas if this seems to make sense.

Selecting the most appropriate strategies is perhaps of greatest importance for total health promotion, since the strategies are the engine room that enables the achievement of greater health.

You might, in the end, come up with something like **Figure 39** (though the outcomes of total health promotion are never entirely predictable).

Note that this figure is not the only health-promoting solution – there are many other ways of promoting autonomy for the adolescent, some of them at least hinted at in the other proposed rational fields. However, at least **Figure 39** respects Matthew, it tries to help him define his own goals, and to conceive of his life situation as realistically as possible. Just as importantly, this foundational rational field approach is disarmingly frank. By bringing together the various salient rational fields it honestly displays a wide range of beyond-the-evidence assumptions, and the health promoter just as honestly displays her own – so treating herself and her subject with serious openness.

THE RATIONAL FIELD TEMPLATE USED FOR INDIVIDUAL THERAPY

Total health promotion may be used as a form of therapy. It is especially useful where a subject's thinking is not as clear as it could be, and therefore total health promotion has an obvious role in what is conventionally described as 'mental health work'.

TWO FURTHER INDIVIDUAL EXAMPLES

The 'boxing champion'

Peter Breggin believes 'many of the symptoms associated with so-called schizophrenia are blatant attempts to compensate for humiliations experienced while growing up'. His understanding of mental illness may be translated, without residue, into rational fields.

Breggin writes:

> Many of the symptoms associated with so-called schizophrenia are blatant attempts to compensate for humiliations experienced while growing up. I'm reminded of the fifteen-year-old frail, frightened boy who came into the hospital declaring that he was a boxing champion. He even could describe his main bouts. His true story was one of being physically abused at home and dominated by bigger boys at school. With regularity, therapists see young men who attempt to bolster their self-esteem by declaring they are somebody extraordinarily important, when deep down they feel humiliated and worthless.[110]

Of course, the frail 15 year old could conceivably be suffering from a brain abnormality that causes grandiose ideas. However, it is at least as conceivable – and infinitely more meaningful – that his rational field and his environment's rational field are so much at odds that something has to give, and of course the boy is infinitely less powerful than his environment. To over-simplify grossly, the situation might be characterised as in **Figures 40** and **41**.

Looked at one way this is nothing more than a paraphrase of Breggin's account of the situation. However, expressing things in this simple format allows a judgement about which (if any) rational field is a problem, allows the assessment of different rational fields, and suggests solutions that involve changing one or more rational fields – and not automatically or necessarily the boy's.

For one example, a total health promotion therapist might decide that the problem with the boy's rational field is the strategy, not the goal, and work on alternative strategies to achieve it. Alternatively, and this would be much more challenging, she might decide to work to change the prevailing environmental rational field, using the general foundations rational field template – hoping to achieve the most healthy school. Perhaps like **Figure 42**.

It no doubt seems quite unrealistic to suggest that the total health promoter should concentrate on the system rather than the individual (after all, it is infinitely easier to make the boy fit the system than the system fit the boy). However, total health promotion must resist conventional assumptions. The basic premise of total health promotion is that we have got our classification systems wrong, or at least that which classification is the most health promoting is an open question. The total health promoter should not prejudge, but should display rational fields as they seem to be, and should work out what could happen given the application of the foundational rational field template.

The whole point of total health promotion is that nothing is fixed in stone and there is everything to play for – after all, health is at stake.

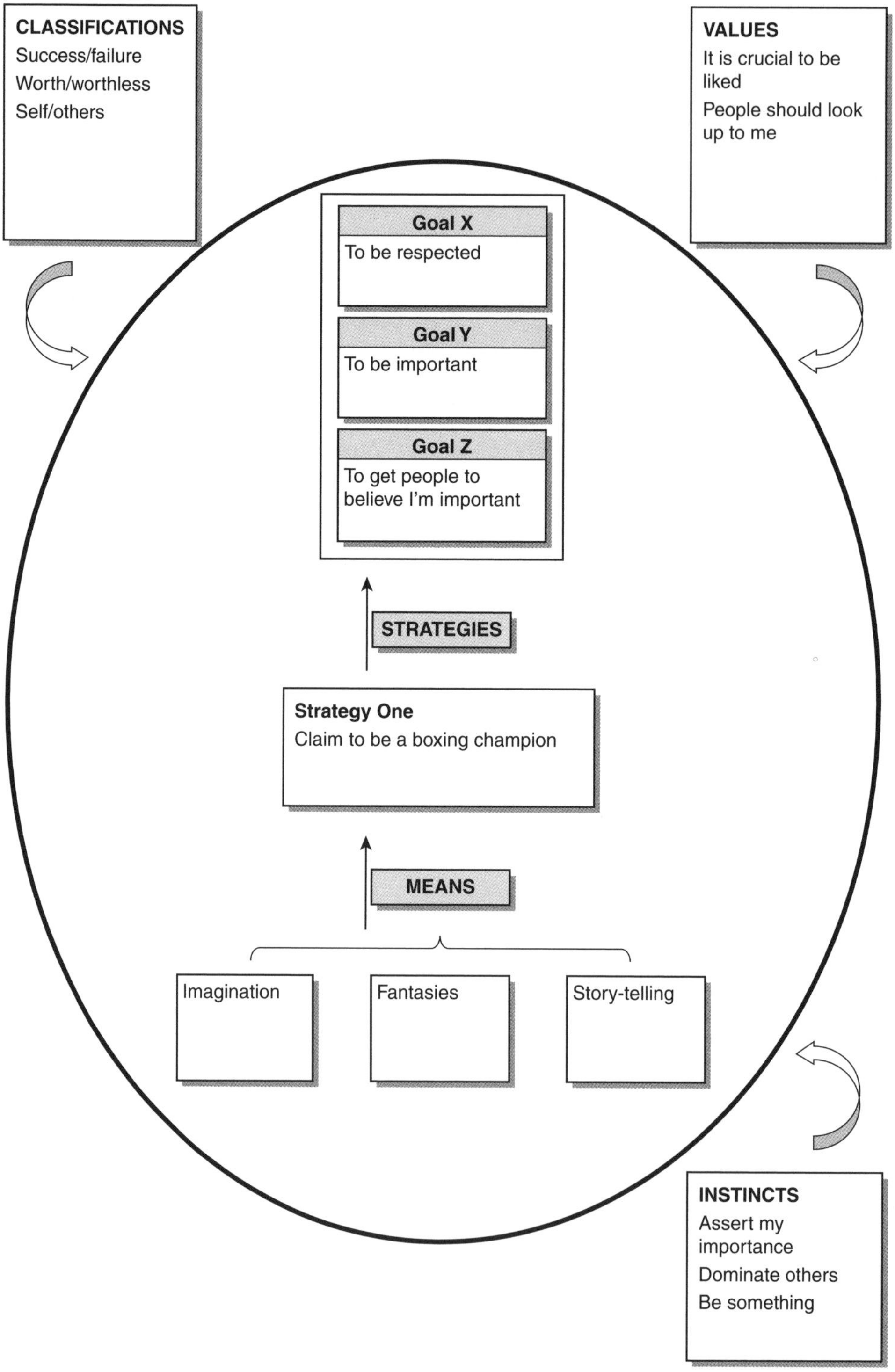

Figure 40 The 'Boxing Champion's' rational field

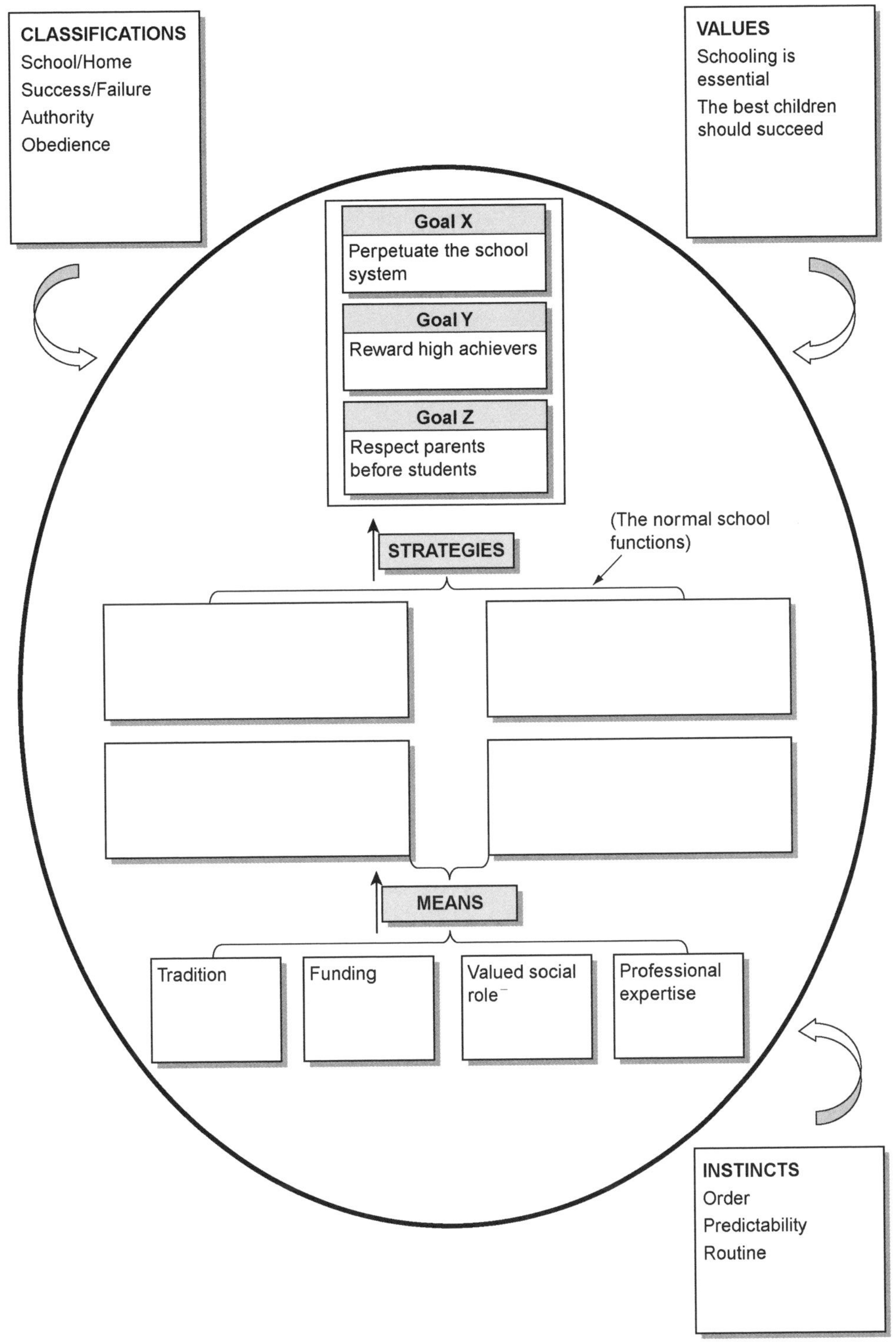

Figure 41 The 'Boxing Champion's' school's prevailing rational field

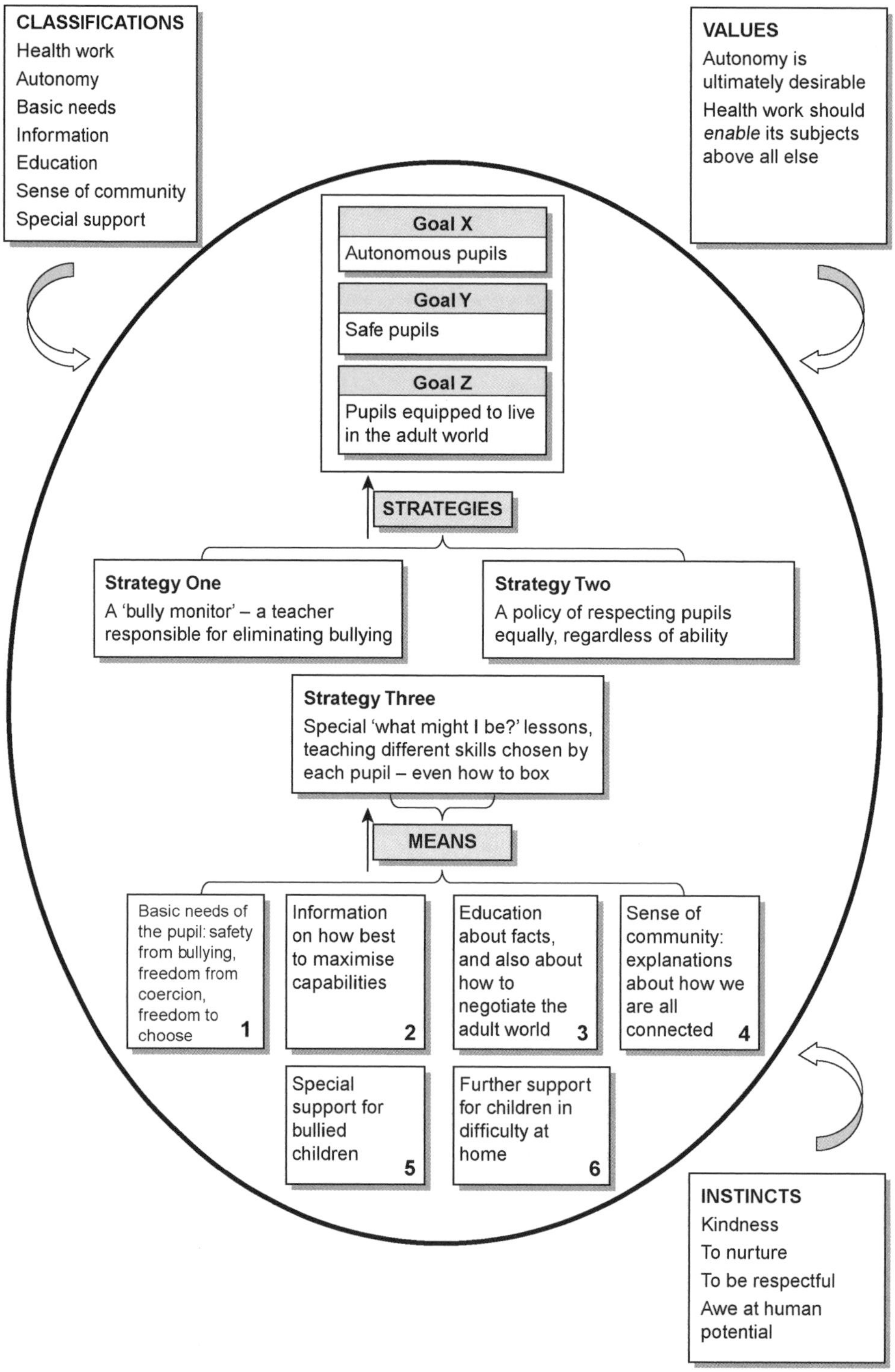

Figure 42 A possible strategy to achieve a healthier school using the General Foundations Rational Field Template

Of course, in reality – at least as things stand – the boy would be seen as the problem, and the total health promoter would probably have to go along with this. But this need not mean colluding with psychiatric classifications and drugs, since these are potentially damaging to the boy (especially the effects of drugs and the effect of being diagnosed with schizophrenia):

> All people suffer from one degree or another of mental helplessness in their routine lives. They need to collect their wits or regain their composure before proceeding with some difficult task. That is, they need to become rational and self-determined, and not helpless, despite their fears.[110]

Another way of putting this is that the total health promoter should help people create rational fields appropriate both to them and to the rational fields that surround them – and then work on making their chosen fields come to pass. Pretending that you are a famous boxer is not a good tactic because it cannot possibly fit within surrounding rational fields. But asking for protection from bullying and developing actual talents – even if they are not immediately valued by surrounding rational fields – is.

Melissa's triumph over anxiety

Breggin also relates the story of Melissa, who suffered paralysing panic attacks:

> Melissa at age twenty-five had an undergraduate degree in accounting and was working as an assistant bookkeeper, a job she found boring and without a future. She also had a boyfriend, an alcoholic who gave her little love and no security. Her true love was laboratory science, but the closest she came to it was looking longingly at a *Scientific American* or *Science News* in her spare time.
>
> Melissa had told her first psychiatrist, 'I'll be sitting at my desk in the library and all of a sudden I'm frightened to death. I've got to get up. I've got to get away from the whole building. But of course, I can't; I work there. Sometimes I'll try to hide in the record room for a while. But it doesn't really matter what I do. I start breathing fast and I can't catch my breath. If I try to stand up, I'll see spots and start to faint.'
>
> ... Melissa's psychiatrist told her that she had a physical problem – a hyperactive nervous system – and he prescribed Valium to 'smooth out the nerves'. But when Melissa got home she decided that drugs couldn't solve her problems, and she looked for another doctor.

Breggin told her she was preoccupied with her apparent problem – the symptoms – rather than her real problem, that she was not in control of her life. Melissa was eventually able to take charge of her destiny, and years later she explained how, to Dr Breggin:

> 'I remember how frightened I used to be about making any choices, and I remember one day how you told me that very few choices in life are irrevocable. I learned that I could make a choice, try it out, and move in another direction if it didn't work out. It wasn't all life and death like my mother said. I could find my way step by step ...
>
> 'Oh, yeah,' she added. 'I had to get out of the victim role. I had to stop feeling that everything unfair on earth was being done to me, and instead that I could actually direct my life. That was why I was able to tell my boyfriend to leave. And why I was able to go back to school.'

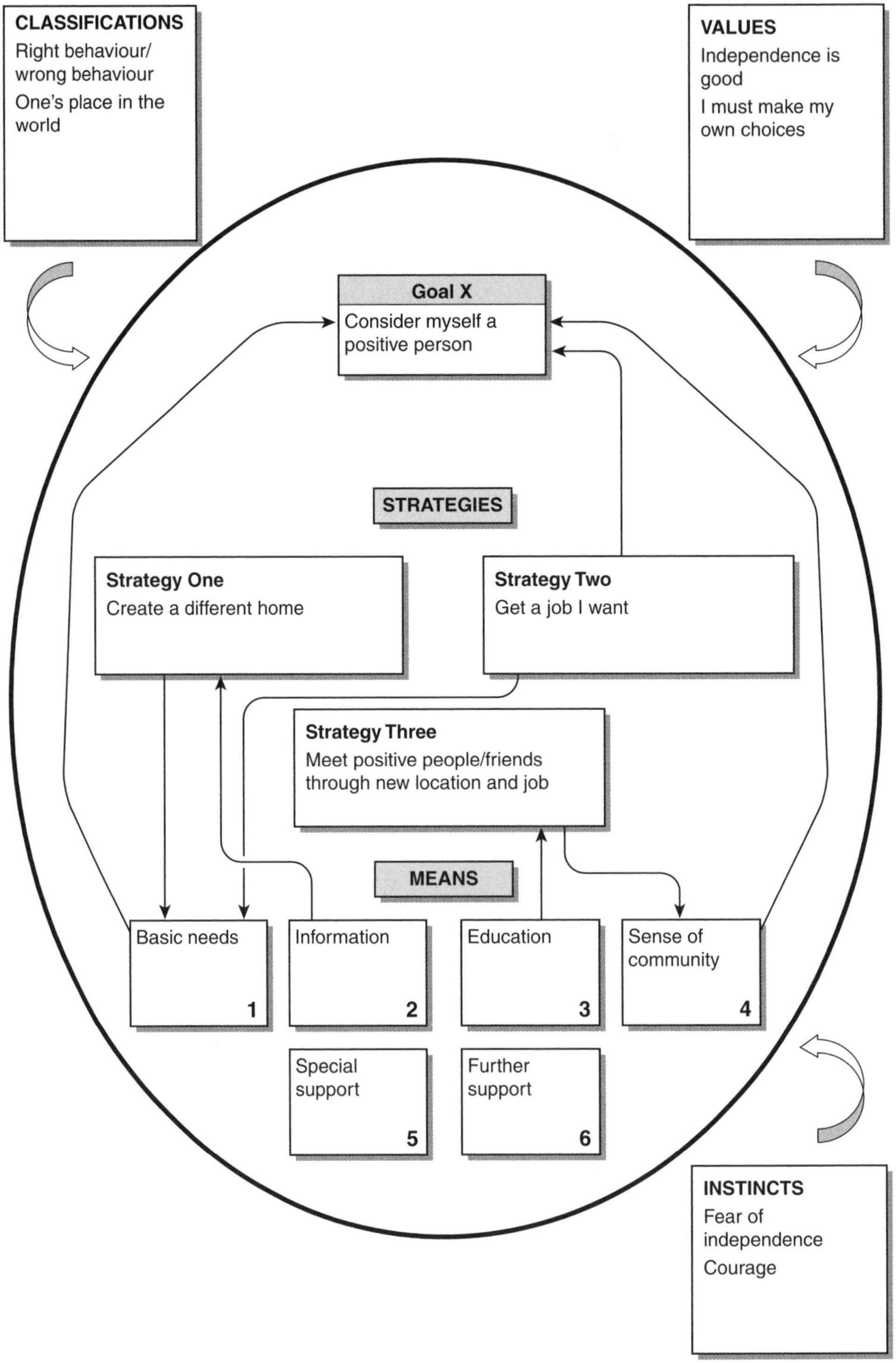

Figure 43 Melissa's healthy rational field

Melissa obtained an advanced degree in science and now works for a respected research institute (see **Figure 43**).

RATIONAL FIELDS AND THE HUMAN EXPERIENCE

If you take the stories of people who have experienced mental trouble – especially those who have been through the psychiatric system – certain conclusions are irresistible:

1. Regardless of whether beyond-the-evidence psychiatric speculations are actually true (and even if *every bit* of a person's illness could be attributed to a brain malfunction) being mentally ill is an experience in which the sufferer continually tries to make sense of what is happening to her.

2. The attempt to make sense of what is happening never happens in a vacuum – it always happens within other rational fields (within a context in which other people have interests, in which institutions have interests, in which there are laws, in which there is culture, normalities of various kinds, and so on).

3. Any attempt to make sense of what is happening to a person cannot succeed if these other rational fields are ignored – such an *in vacuo* understanding is quite obviously unrealistic (unfortunately it is a common psychiatric approach).

4. Equally, chemical, surgical or electrical therapy cannot possibly ultimately succeed if these other rational fields (and the rational fields of the person herself) are ignored, since the person must go on after the therapy to rehabilitate or recover.

5. People obviously strive toward the creation of rational fields, since this is what gives meaning to their suffering.

There are countless books written by ex-psychiatric patients that testify to this.[51] Denise's story is typical:

Denise's story

> When I was younger I was suicidal because nobody could hear what I was saying and I felt desperate. I went into hospital when I was sixteen and had a very difficult experience with all sorts of diagnoses and all sorts of medication. Right through my school years and adolescence I was being referred to psychiatrists. So it was always there. And I had severe behavioral problems at school.
>
> I asked for help in every way that I could. When I had nowhere else to turn, suicide was my best option because I just couldn't tolerate the feelings I had. It wasn't that I actually wanted to die, but after I had been in the public health system, my spirit was broken. It changed to the point where I wanted to die and that was very different for me.

Translated into rational fields, there were obviously massively conflicting fields at play in Denise's life, not least Denise's own rational field and the rational fields of the prevailing system.

> I had problems on and off over the next ten years, but managed to hide them. I felt I needed to hide them from my work, from whatever. I would go away for six months but

> manage to stay on the job roster so it didn't look like there were gaps in my CV. Somehow I could cover them up.

This was an inappropriate rational strategy. It was not positive personally, and it could never mesh with the external rational fields that surround Denise.

> After a few days I managed to get out of isolation, into the main ward. In the main ward, we were locked into the dorms. There was a woman lying there in full light – there was a light outside all the windows so you couldn't get any darkness or peace at night, but this woman was lying there masturbating, which was quite frightening for me at that stage. There were no doors on the toilets, and the men and women used the same area at times. Everybody had to have showers at the same time, so they'd use one shower, and all the women would go in, and then all the men would go in. I felt very unsafe that there were no doors on the toilets. I certainly didn't want to go into the toilet. They shepherded people from one room to another so that everybody was in the same place at the same time.
>
> You had to go outside for three hours at a time, if that's what they wanted you to do, whether it was raining or whatever. There was a ten-foot wire fence enclosing the ward and a recreation area. We were caged in. You couldn't sit down and watch TV or read a book. There was nothing to read in the ward. When we were locked all together in the lounge area, there was a women's toilet in the lounge, but there was no lock on the door. It could open and you were just sitting there on the toilet in front of a whole room of men and women. And I had no access to any of my own clothes.
>
> When I was in an isolation lounge, there was this one guy that I could see through a glass door and he could see me. He was drooling, he was tied in a straitjacket; this is only four years ago, he was in a straitjacket. He was drooling – so drugged he could hardly move. And we both just sort of reached out. There was a real connection, like people that were being tortured.
>
> The other thing that really freaked me out was this fire alarm went off, and all the nurses disappeared to see what it was. I was locked in a room for about ten minutes with the whole window covered in smoke. I had no way of getting out. That was incredibly frightening.
>
> It's taken me a long time to talk about it to a point where I can say a lot of what happened. It was really that the staff were so abusive and I was totally under their control. There was nothing that I could have done. Unless you have ever had that experience you could never, ever convey what it felt like. The powerlessness.

Any possibility of Denise expressing her rational field was crushed by the oppressive rational field of the prevailing system.

> The first time I began to receive appropriate treatment and started to recover was when I got to Ashburn Hall. This is also where my artwork starts. The first process that was helpful in my recovery is reflected in my art therapy. It was the beginning steps. After that first art therapy session, I just wanted to paint. I wanted to get it down. I wanted to get it out. I wanted to explain what was going on.

At last an appropriate rational field seemed possible to Denise. It came into being because the dominant system's rational field allowed it.

> One problem that I have is poor impulse control. Before, if somebody had pissed me off, I would have whacked them. I just had no concept that what I did actually had any effect on anybody.
>
> Now I do have that awareness. That developed from being in Ashburn Hall with other people. I was in groups where people were saying, Well, this is what you have done and

> this is how it has affected me. It helped me to develop an understanding of what I did. So now if somebody pisses me off, I have much greater choice of what I can do. ...
>
> To know that I can actually live through the ending of the relationship is important because my depression is very tied up with loss, which is very tied up with death.[51]

Denise has begun to recognise the components of her rational field, and is learning to identify positive and negative aspects.

You understand troubled people – and they understand themselves – by exploring rational fields. Call it what you will, this is the reality of it. To deny it – to think that your rational field is the only truly rational field, or to think that your rational field is perfectly value-free – is to condemn troubled people to endless further trouble: it is to perpetuate bafflement in people who are finding life difficult (why are my rational fields utterly worthless and why are yours utterly valuable?).

All this may seem over-simple. I imagine it does to people who are used to complicated and elaborate technicalities and diagnostic systems. But making things simple is an asset, not a problem. Of course the world is complicated – too complicated for us to grasp without our artificial classifications, but we can understand it in very human ways, and the best way to do so is to capture the essence of our situations, which is precisely what the use of rational field interpretations is meant to do.

It is quite possible to create very complex and extensive rational fields – and sometimes this may be necessary – but mostly it is enough for us to have a clear and basic grasp of what is wrong – then we can set about doing something about it with clear sight.

MORE COMPLEX HEALTH PROMOTION TASKS – THE IMMUNISATION ISSUE

Naturally, total health promotion is useful beyond individual therapy – it wouldn't be *total* health promotion if it were not.

IMMUNISATION – SIMPLE

There is an establishment view of immunisation that can be found in numerous government publications and websites.[132] This can be summarised as a very simple rational field, using the rational field template shown in **Figure 44**.

Sometimes people have false beliefs about immunisation (these may or may not be irrational, dependent upon the structure of their reasoning[104]). Mrs Jones has a false belief – she thinks the second Mumps, Measles and Rubella (MMR) immunisation has a 10% risk of causing brain damage in her daughter, and therefore has decided against accepting it. Her current rational field looks like that depicted in **Figure 45**.

The health promotion task in this case is simple, though it is not merely a question of explaining that Mrs Jones's strategy is based on false information. Rather it is a

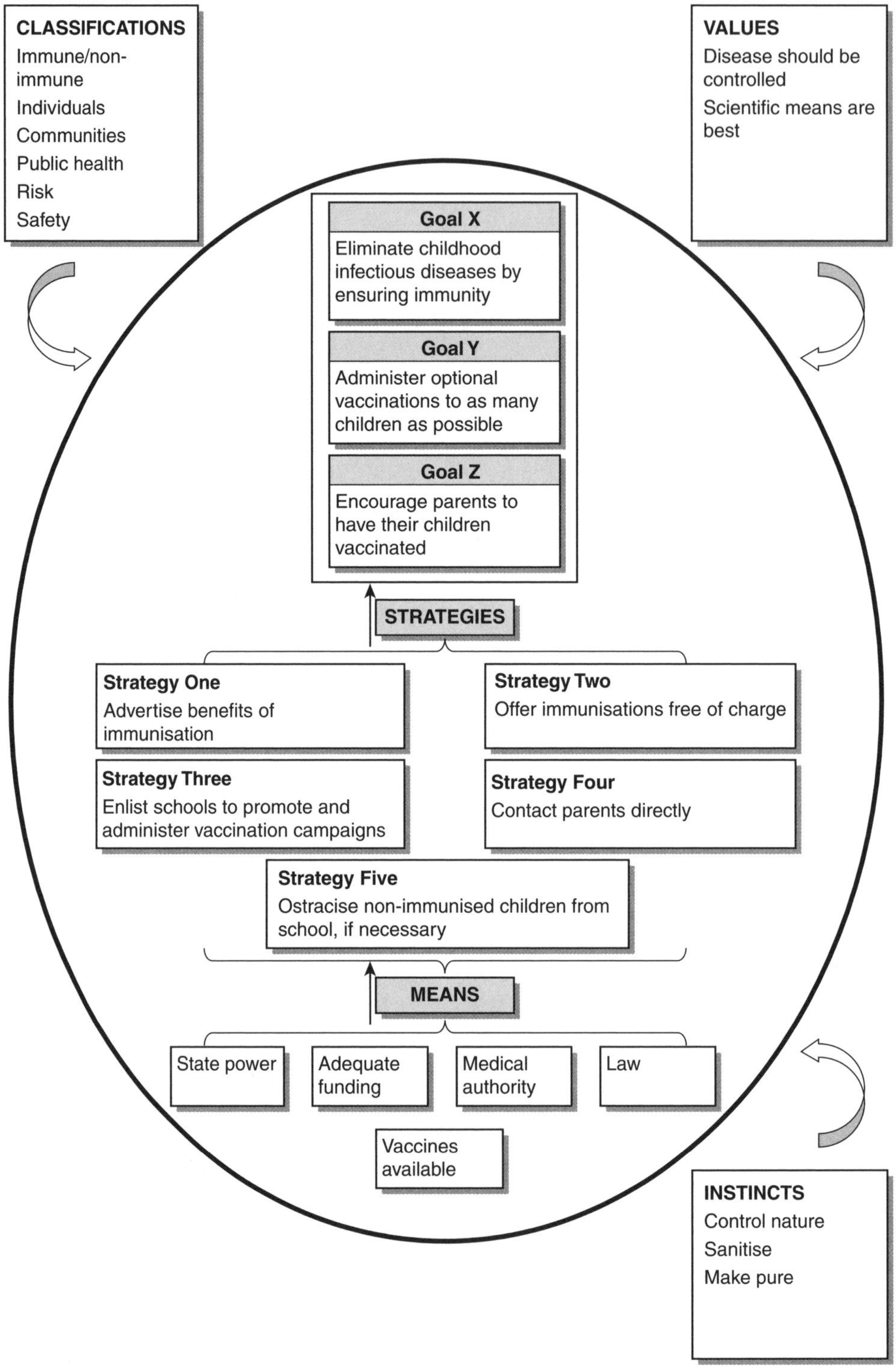

Figure 44 The conventional view of childhood immunisation

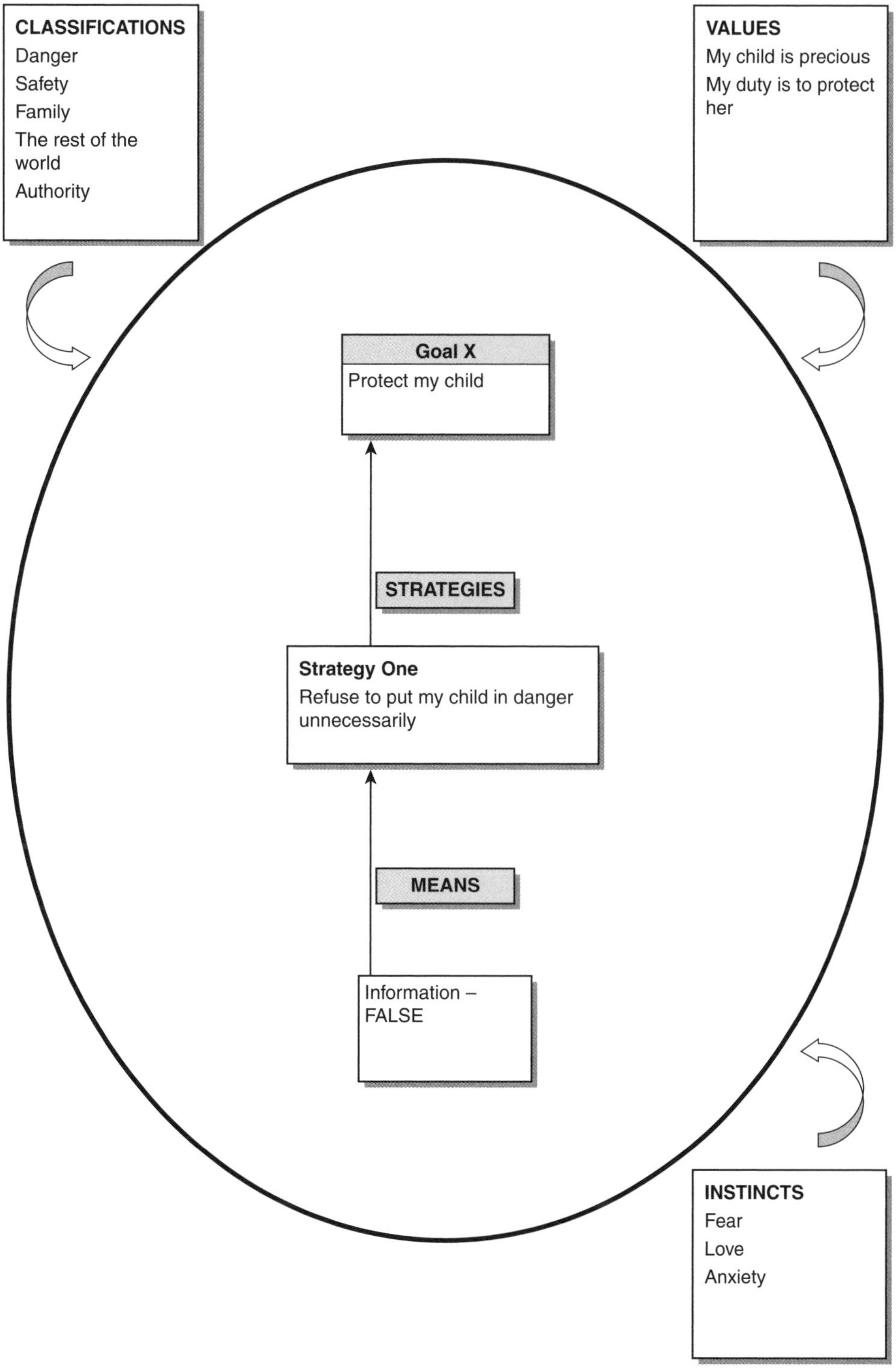

Figure 45 Mrs Jones's 'false belief' rational field

question of presenting the evidence *within an honest rational field*. So, the total health promoter must explain the establishment rational field – explaining its value source, its evidence and its logic (this is relatively easy to do with the help of the simple rational field illustrated in **Figure 43**.) He should also explain a summary rational field for the anti-immunisation movement.[133]

Then he must present Mrs Jones's rational field in the same way, including her false belief about risk – and compare the three (he can do this verbally, but preferably he will do it visually – it will soon be possible for him to do this by means of computer technology[134]). What the total health promoter cannot do – and this is another way in which total health promotion is radically different from conventional health promotion – is to present one rational field only, or *convince* the subject to favour one rational field ahead of the other. Total health promotion seeks as a priority to promote autonomy – and promoting autonomy means informing and educating subjects as openly as possible.

IMMUNISATION – MORE COMPLEX

Now imagine a troubled Mrs Jones returning to the health promoter. She tells him, 'I was going to have Madison [her daughter] immunised with MMR, but then I read this at the official website':

> [Note: quoted directly from the website – not edited to eliminate repetition.]
>
> The first dose of the MMR vaccine protects at least 90% of children against measles, at least 90% against mumps, and at least 95% against rubella.
>
> **Why does my child need a second dose?**
>
> **Question 6**
>
> 1000 children all offered the first dose of the MMR vaccine
> 900 accept 810 PROTECTED(81% of children)
> 190 NOT PROTECTED(19% of children)
> 90 NOT PROTECTED against measles
> 100 do not accept = NOT PROTECTED
> Vaccine works in 90%
> Vaccine does not work in 10%
>
> In at least 10% of children who receive one dose of MMR, it does not work against the measles virus. The figure is 10% for mumps, and 5% for rubella. In addition, about 10% of children do not receive the first dose of the MMR vaccine, for various reasons (e.g. missed appointment). Thus, with nearly 20% of children still vulnerable to measles, outbreaks would occur. These would involve older children and infants under one year (when measles results in more complications) and those with reduced immunity (those who cannot have MMR vaccine and have to rely on everyone else's immunity for their protection).
>
> The chance of your child not being protected against measles after one dose of MMR is around 1 in 10. After two doses the chance of your child not being protected against measles falls to around 1 in 100, i.e. 99% protection. The second dose also gives children who missed the first dose another chance to be vaccinated.
>
> Blood tests to check immunity before giving a second dose or targeting only non-recipients are not recommended because there are drawbacks. The risk of side-effects is 10 times

> lower with a second dose of MMR vaccine. On an individual level, for at least 10% of children who receive one dose of MMR, it does not provide protection against measles. The figure is approximately 10% for mumps, and 5% for rubella. In addition, about 10% of children do not receive the first dose of the MMR vaccine, for various reasons (e.g. missed appointment). These groups therefore remain susceptible after only one dose of the MMR vaccine has been offered. On a community level, it is impossible to achieve 'population protection' (herd immunity), and therefore effective disease control, using a one-dose schedule. For example, if 90% of children receive a dose of MMR, and in 10% of these the vaccine fails to work, only 81% will be immune after one dose. However, more than 90% of the population needs to be immune for measles to be eliminated. If 'population protection' is not achieved, breakthrough outbreaks will occur. Cases will occur among non-recipients, non-responders and infants aged less than one year (who are too young to have the vaccine). Children who are immunocompromised, in whom MMR vaccine is contraindicated, and in whom measles has a high fatality, will also be at risk. This has been the experience in the USA, which saw large breakthrough outbreaks in the early 1990s, resulting in 55,000 cases and over 100 deaths. In a setting where the level of population immunity is high, but not high enough to achieve 'population protection', outbreaks will tend to affect older children. If, for example, 81% of children are immune after one dose, the circulation of wild measles virus is interrupted to the extent that the children who remain susceptible have a reduced chance of being exposed to it during early childhood. With time, a growing number of non-immune, older children will accumulate. Eventually, there will be enough of them to allow epidemics to occur. Even when indigenous measles is eliminated, imported cases may still occur and UK children may be exposed abroad and by returning travellers. Maintaining the highest possible level of population immunity is therefore vital. A second MMR vaccination protects most children who do not respond to the first dose: around 90% will have a good response to the second dose. The chance of an individual remaining susceptible is reduced from 1 in 10 to around 1 in 100 after a second dose.
>
> By offering a second dose of MMR vaccine, those children who did not even receive the first dose get a second chance. A further benefit is that it boosts the antibodies of children who did respond to the first dose. A two-dose schedule is the only strategy that will eliminate measles in the UK. If only non-recipients were targeted the 10% of children that have received the first dose, but have not responded to it, would remain susceptible. Mass antibody testing and recall of non-immune children would be difficult to implement, and would add greatly to the cost of the measles vaccination programme. Serum antibody testing would mean taking a blood sample from four year-olds – an invasive procedure that is traumatic for a young child. The test is not 100% accurate and it would fail to identify some susceptible children, who would consequently not receive a further dose of MMR, and who would therefore remain at risk.[135]

Despite the awkward writing style, this sums up the official reasoning very well. However, the task of the total health promoter is to expose the rational field as it actually is – not just as the officials want it to look. And this means setting it out using the rational field template – exposing its beyond-the-evidence assumptions and its value source (see **Figure 46**). It also means laying it alongside alternative rational fields, including the clearest representation of Mrs Jones's rational field (decided in collaboration with Mrs Jones). The task of the rational health promoter is not to take anything at face value – to take neither Mrs Jones nor the official rational field as absolute.

If Mrs Jones then decides that she would like her child to have a blood test rather than the MMR booster the total health promoter should lay out a redesigned rational field for Mrs Jones, check it for logic and internal consistency, and then lay it out against surrounding fields (including **Figure 46**), enabling Mrs Jones to reflect on the likely consequences of her decision.

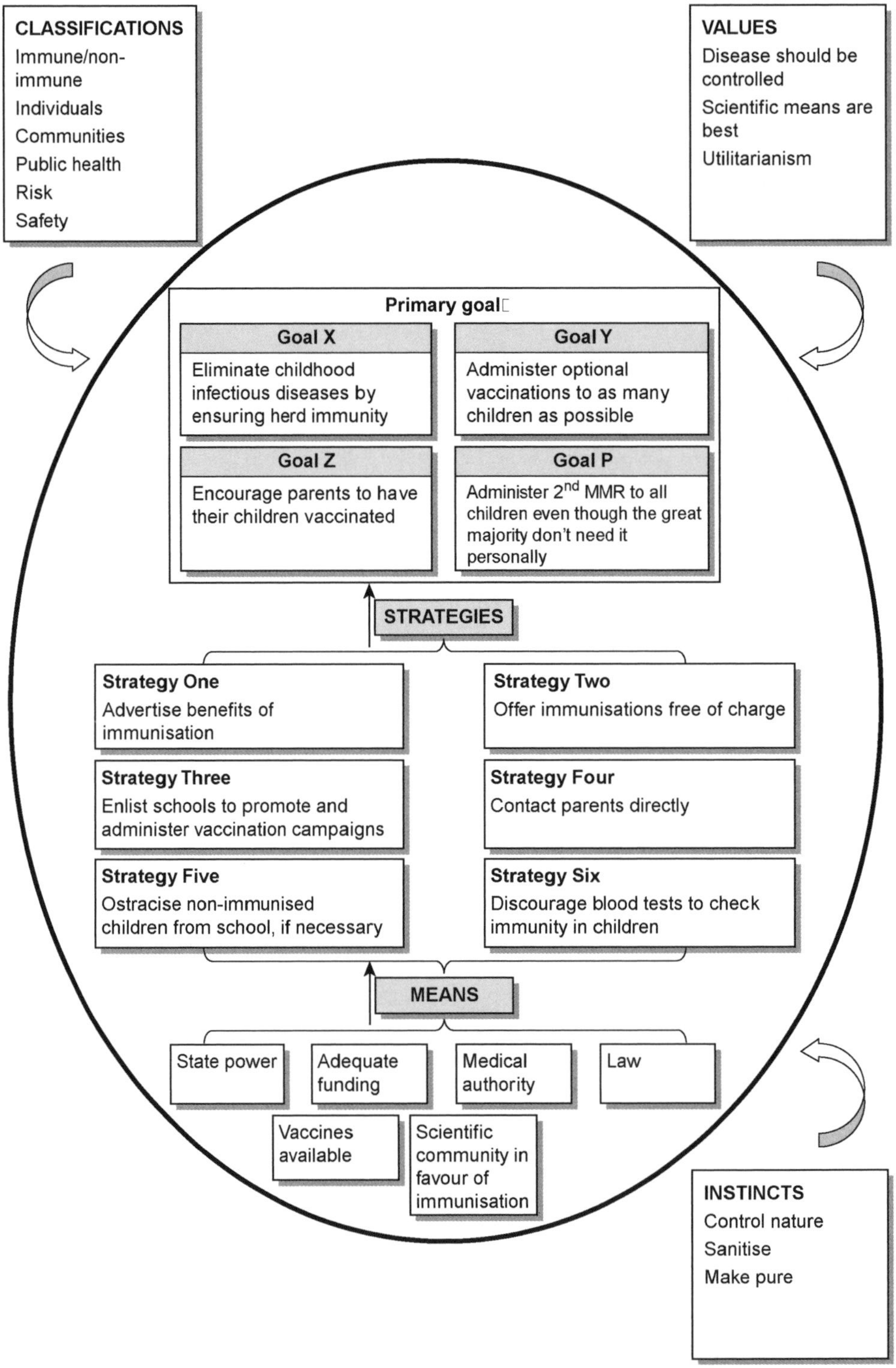

Figure 46 The conventional view of childhood immunisation more fully expressed

TOTAL HEALTH PROMOTION AND POLICY SETTING

The examples so far have illustrated how the total health promoter might work with individuals in therapy and to help them decide on strategy when they are not ill. It is possible to work with groups in just the same fashion – by filling in the **general foundations rational field template** given in **Figure 37**. Instead of individual goals the total health promoter simply needs to ascertain and spell out group goals – and to do the same with strategies and means. For example, a family might be wondering what best to do for an elderly and increasingly frail parent – and in this case rational fields designed both for key individuals and various groups would be extremely clarifying.

It is also possible to use the rational field template to assess health promotion policy in general. For example, the rational field template might be applied to conventional health promotion targets (for example, the **38 Targets for Health in the European Region**[136]). These might be simply specified and assessed internally for logic, and their walls (their values and classifications) revealed. The fields for different targets could then be compared in a similar fashion. Do they fit together? Are they inspired by the same values? After that the '**38 Target**' fields could be compared with surrounding fields – for example, a selection of general life rational fields of typical members of the target population (to see how realistic the **38 Targets** are, in relation to people's usual aspirations). Finally these rational fields could be compared with other ways of spending taxpayers' money – and the results could be published openly for general debate and agreement or disagreement from the target population. (The total health promoter trusts people to make their own judgements. The conventional health promoter lives in continual fear that the public will make the 'wrong' decision, and so rarely gives us any choice at all about population strategies.)

TOTAL HEALTH PROMOTION IS RADICAL HEALTH PROMOTION

The above examples and solutions have been fairly conventional, so as not to alienate interested conventional health promoters. However, be in no doubt that total health promotion is meant to challenge conventional certainties head on. It is open to the total health promoter to come up with *any* rational field in response to any given situation, so long as he is aiming to promote autonomy. He does not have to be bound by the usual medical priorities. Anything goes for the total health promoter.

For example, if the total health promoter wants to assess the rationality and autonomy-creation prowess of current establishment health promotion, he can display the prevailing field and compare it with any alternative he knows of or can imagine.

Let's say he is feeling a little mischievous one day. So he takes out a **general foundations rational field template** and begins to fill it in as in **Figure 47**.

Who knows, **Figure 47** might work better than our present arrangement. No one knows that it wouldn't, and it certainly fits better with foundational health values than conventional ways of promoting health.

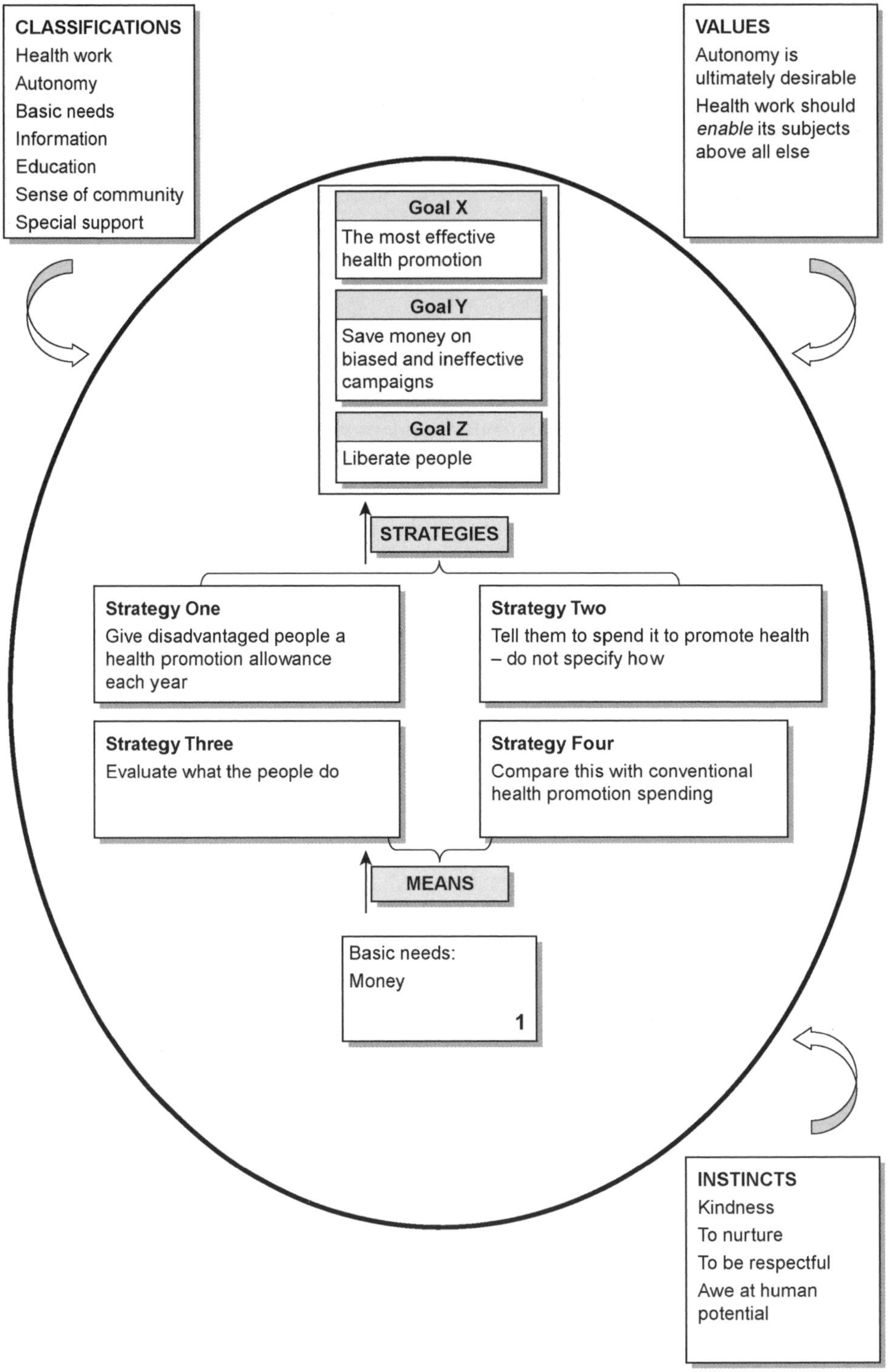
CLASSIFICATIONS
Health work
Autonomy
Basic needs
Information
Education
Sense of community
Special support
VALUES
Autonomy is ultimately desirable
Health work should *enable* its subjects above all else
Goal X
The most effective health promotion
Goal Y
Save money on biased and ineffective campaigns
Goal Z
Liberate people
STRATEGIES
Strategy One
Give disadvantaged people a health promotion allowance each year
Strategy Two
Tell them to spend it to promote health – do not specify how
Strategy Three
Evaluate what the people do
Strategy Four
Compare this with conventional health promotion spending
MEANS
Basic needs:
Money
1
INSTINCTS
Kindness
To nurture
To be respectful
Awe at human potential

Figure 47 Promote health by giving the people the money usually granted to conventional health promotion Institutes

THE BENEFITS OF TOTAL HEALTH PROMOTION

Total health promotion determinedly resists entrapment within the walls of parochial rational fields. Total health promotion is revolutionary health promotion. The total health promoter does not exclusively promote simplistic, rigid rational fields like – you should stop smoking, you should immunise your child, you should get on your bike, you shouldn't drink, etc. It is not surprising that these techniques don't work[137] because they are abstracted from and alien to the sea of rational fields we all inhabit.

TWENTY BENEFITS OF TOTAL HEALTH PROMOTION

1. Total health promotion is open and honest. Because total health promoters must complete rational field templates as they plan to promote health, their thinking is revealed – both to the health promoters themselves and to anyone else given access to the template.

2. Total health promotion openly acknowledges that there are no absolutely right answers in health promotion.

3. Total health promotion recognises that the world is fundamentally interconnected and that therefore a focus on a particular rational field can only ever be part of the story.

4. Total health promotion asks both promoters and recipients to try to understand and to reveal the instincts, values and classifications that inform their choosing and planning. In so doing it explodes the myth that health promotion is value-free, and that health is a supreme value that requires no more elucidation.

By using the rational field template, total health promotion exposes the walls that surround any rational field. This can come as a surprise to those who are used to thinking that their particular rational field is all there is, but then this is the primary value of rational fields. Thinking and planning using rational fields is essentially an exercise in remedial philosophical education for people obsessed with their own importance, and fixated with the conviction that their way of getting through life is the true and only way to do it.

5. Total health promotion provides a means of scrutinising the rationality of health promotion plans, by assessing the relationship between means, strategies and goals. The rational field template sets out the plan systematically and so allows the testing of logic, coherence, likely benefit, likely cost, and so on (more sophisticated analyses may be built onto the template as required).

This method also enables the evaluation of goals, and assists in assessing the match between selected goals and surrounding instincts, classifications and values.

6. Total health promotion uses an explicit and thoroughly argued theoretical base – the foundations theory of health. This is in stark contrast to conventional

health promotion, which merely assumes that health is good, and that any way to bring about more of it must therefore be acceptable.

7. Total health promotion is the *quest for autonomy*. The justification for acting on any completed rational field template must be that the plan maximises opportunity for its subject(s).

8. In order for health promoters to maximise opportunity for subjects they have to know what the subjects' goals and interests are, so they have to ask them – thus involving them directly in health promotion.

9. The rational field template need not be used by health promoters alone – health promotion is not an activity that is exclusive to a particular sort of person or professional group. Anyone can do it and anyone may be involved in it.

10. Rational field templates can and should be widely distributed and completed. This is a perfect way to find out what sort of health the general public really wants.

11. Total health promotion takes people seriously. By use of the rational field template, it seeks always to understand them and their goals, means and strategies. It understands that all of us are rational fields, that we are made up of rational fields, and that we live surrounded by a sea of rational fields.

12. Total health promotion avoids artificial categories like 'responsible', 'irresponsible', 'unhealthy behaviour', 'risky behaviour' and so on. Not only are such classifications gross over-simplifications of a world teeming with rationality, but they inevitably and radically restrict the focus of what might be done to help create more autonomy for people.

13. Rational field templates may be used as a form of therapy when people experience life difficulties.

14. Rational field templates may be used to help formulate clear, efficient and health-promoting management plans if a person is diseased.

15. Total health promotion tries to avoid those artificial classifications that inhibit autonomy promotion. This means, for example, that total health promotion does not distinguish absolutely between the physical, social and mental – these supposedly different spheres are never its first focus. Rather the question is always: *how can I promote autonomy in this complex situation*? Almost without fail the use of the rational field template produces an intermeshed plan, a plan in which the mental, physical and social are part of each other.

16. Additional analysis and practical work is often required in total health promotion. This book has merely offered a sketch of the basic skeleton of total health promotion. There are related techniques available that may usefully complement the rational field template. For example, the Ethical Grid, the Rings of Uncertainty and the Autonomy Test.[98] These and other visually-based ethical decision-making methods are currently being developed into a semi-intelligent decision-making package for use in health work, and it is hoped that they may become widely adopted.[134]

There are also many quantitative techniques available (in economics, for example) and these may be needed for complex or large-scale rational field analyses.

17. Total health promotion is itself a rational field, swimming in a sea of rational fields. Like any other manufactured idea, total health promotion has its own instincts, classifications and values. But this is not a problem, since all rational fields have their perimeters. Indeed it is a benefit, since its beyond-the-evidence basis can be perfectly known to all total health promoters and their subjects (or at least as well-known as human insight and honesty permit).

18. Rational field theory reveals a 'shadowy pattern of truth'.[100] The idea seems, in utter crudity, to say something about the way the world really is – an unbelievably complex set of purposive systems.

19. Rational field theory explains why we have so much trouble in reaching agreement about human affairs in general. When we disagree, we disagree for all manner of biological, psychological and cultural reasons. The rational field idea is a very useful way to lay out our disagreements, so that we can see clearly what it is that we disagree about: have different members of an ethics committee, for instance, complete rational field templates about any given issue, and all verbal manoeuvring and subterfuge will evaporate like the dew at daybreak – a clear set of goals, strategies and means, and an honest explanation of their source in beyond-the-evidence, makes disputes instantly transparent.

20. Rational field theory enables us all to stand back – to ask 'what sorts of rational fields do we really want'? The theme of this book has been that nothing is as fixed as it seems. Of course much of the world **just is**, whether we like it or not, and there are innumerable natural rational fields that we cannot possibly escape (the ageing of our bodies' systems for example). However, we most certainly do not have to add to this grinding inevitability by creating permanently fixed categories of our own.

Total Health Promotion has used the example of psychiatry, since psychiatry is very obviously a social disaster of our own making. But there are countless other questionable rational fields around us – no manufactured rational field has to be set in stone forever. If rational fields are not promoting as much autonomy for all of us as they might then we should change them. Obviously, I realise how hard it is to do this. But I submit that one of the reasons it is so hard is that most of us cannot yet conceive of the impermanent nature of our rational fields. And we do change our systems, usually very slowly. If we can at least *begin* to understand and apply the rational field idea then perhaps we can speed things up a bit.

Note: One way of conceiving of what happened to the Heavenly Creatures is to think of them as inhabiting a shared and shattered rational field. As they killed Honora Parker its walls collapsed completely (as the values that held the field together became horribly apparent). And immediately, new rational fields (one for each girl) emerged.

CONCLUSION

As with all my books, I find that I began the investigation in what I thought was ignorance, and yet I end it not only stating what seems obvious, but stating something I knew to be obvious all along. Thus the only real value I can find in my work is that at least I make the effort to express the steps clearly – that is, I try to show the *structure of the obvious*. And having done this, at least it becomes possible to plan for practice in theoretical clarity – without falling into the trap of believing that half-examined assumptions are correct or the best.

What is better: that we walk blindly within rational fields, wearing blindfolds of our own making, unwilling and unable to see over the rational fields' walls; or that we are able to detect, develop creatively and select from all manner of rational fields in the continual quest to create autonomy?

References

1. Gurr, Thomas and Cox, H. H. (1957). *Famous Australasian Crimes*, Muller, London, pp. 148–67.
2. *Sun-Star*, Christchurch, New Zealand, 23 August 1954.
3. Furneaux, Rupert (1955). *Famous Criminal Cases*, Vol 2, Wingate, London, pp. 32–49.
4. Hume, D. (1978). *A Treatise of Human Nature*, ed. L. A. Selby-Bigge, Oxford University Press.
5. Reznek, L. (1997). *Evil or Ill?* Routledge, London.
6. Szasz, T. (1997). *Insanity: The Idea and Its Consequences*, Syracuse University Press (Reprint).
7. Polanyi, M. (1958). *Personal Knowledge*, Routledge and Kegan Paul, London.
8. Martin, J. (2000). *The English Legal System*, 2nd edn, Hodder and Stoughton Educational, London.
9. Gavey, N. (1997). In the Name of Science (A commentary on 'Memory Repression and Recovery: What is the Evidence?'). *Health Care Analysis: Journal of Health Philosophy and Practice* **5**, 2.
10. Ereshefsky, M. (ed.) (1992). *The Units of Evolution: Essays on the Nature of the Species*, MIT Press, Cambridge, MA.
11. Blakely, R. J. (1996). *Potential Theory in Gravity and Magnetic Applications*, Cambridge University Press, Cambridge.
12. Guterson, David (1993). *Family Matters: Why Homeschooling Makes Sense*, Harcourt Brace, Harvest edn, p. 177.
13. Cohen, Peter (2000). Is the addiction doctor the voodoo priest of the Western man? Extended version of an article that appeared in *Addiction Research*, Special Issue, **8**, 6. See: wysiwyg://8http://www.cedro-uva.org/lib/cohen.addiction.html
14. http://www.gallup.com/poll/releases/pr010608.asp
15. http://www.religioustolerance.org/chr_exor.htm#pro
16. Bush Calls for Day of Prayer: The text of President Bush's proclamation 13 September, calling for a national day of prayer and remembrance (White House, 13 September 2001) http://www.foxnews.com/story/0,2933,34338,00.html
17. *Sun-Star*, Christchurch, New Zealand, 30 August 1954, p. 4.
18. http://www.januarymagazine.com/profiles/perry.html
19. http://nz.com/NZ/Queer/history/Parker&Hulme.html
20. http://library.christchurch.org.nz/Heritage/ParkerHulme/document.asp
21. US Department of Health and Human Services (1999). *Mental Health: A Report of the Surgeon General*, US Department of Health and Human Services, Substance Abuse and Mental Health Services Administration, Center for Mental Health Services, National Institutes of Health, National Institute of Mental Health, Washington, DC.
22. Kessler, R. C. et al. (1998). A Methodology for Estimating the 12-Month Prevalence of Serious Mental Illness. In *Mental Health, United States*, ed. R. W. Manderscheid and M. J. Henderson, Center for Mental Health Services, pp. 99–109.
23. Regier D. A. et al. (1993). The de facto Mental and Addictive Disorders Service System. Epidemiologic Catchment Area Prospective One Year Prevalence Rate of Disorders and Services. *Archives of General Psychiatry*, **50**(2), 85–94.
24. Manderscheid, R. W. and Sonnerschein, M. A. (1992). *Mental Health in the United States*. US Department of Health and Human Services, Washington, DC.
25. Center for Mental Health Services (1998). *Survey of Mental Health Organizations and General Mental Health Services*. Center for Mental Health Services, Washington, DC.

26. Federal Task Force on Homelessness and Severe Mental Illness (1992). *Outcasts on Main Street: A Report of the Federal Task Force on Homelessness and Severe Mental Illness*, Government Printing Office, Washington, DC.
27. http://www.nami.org/fact.htm (National Alliance for the Mentally Ill (**NAMI**))
28. http://www.mentalwellness.com/referenc/knowledg/schizop.htm
29. Breggin, P. R. (1994). *Toxic Psychiatry*, St. Martin's Press, New York, pp. 94–5.
30. Breggin, P. R. (1994). *Toxic Psychiatry*, St. Martin's Press, New York, pp. 110–12.
31. Walton, Jo Ann (1999). On Living With Schizophrenia, in I. Mudjas and J. Walton (eds), *Nursing and the Experience of Illness*, Routledge, London, pp. 105–6.
32. Andreasen, N. C. (1999). Understanding the causes of schizophrenia. *New England Journal of Medicine*, **340** (Feb. 25), 645.
33. Breggin, P. R. (1994). *Toxic Psychiatry*, St. Martin's Press, New York, p. 13.
34. Jones, P. and Murray, R. M. (1991). The genetics of schizophrenia is the genetics of neurodevelopment. *British Journal of Psychiatry*, **158**, 615–23.
35. Breggin, P. R. (1994). *Toxic Psychiatry*, St. Martin's Press, New York, pp. 33–4.
36. Andreasen, N. C., Paradiso, S. and O'Leary, D. S. (1998). 'Cognitive dysmetria' as an integrative theory of schizophrenia: a dysfunction in cortical-subcortical-cerebellar circuitry? *Schizophrenia Bulletin*, **24**, 203–18.
37. Woods, B. T. (1998). Is schizophrenia a progressive neurodevelopmental disorder? Toward a unitary pathogenetic mechanism. *American Journal of Psychiatry*, **155**, 1661–70.
38. Armstrong, E., Schleicher, A., Omran, H., Curtis, M. and Zilles, K. (1995). The ontogeny of human gyrification. *Cerebral Cortex*, **5**, 56–63.
39. Popper, K. (1969). *Conjectures and Refutations* (5th edn), Routledge, London.
40. Andreasen, N. C. (1997). Linking mind and brain in the study of mental illness: a project for a scientific psychopathology. *Science*, **275**, 1586–93.
41. Braff, D. L. (1993). Information processing and attention dysfunctions in schizophrenia. *Schizophrenia Bulletin*, **19**, 233–59.
42. Breggin, P. R. (1994). *Toxic Psychiatry*, St. Martin's Press, New York, pp. 112–13.
43. Mortensen, P. B., Pedersen, C. B., Westergaard, T., et al. (1999). Effects of family history and place and season of birth on the risk of schizophrenia. *New England Journal of Medicine*, **340**, 603–8.
44. Moldin, S. O. and Gottesman, I. (1997). At issue: genes, experience, and chance in schizophrenia – positioning for the 21st century. *Schizophrenia Bulletin*, **23**, 547–61.
45. Breggin, P. R. (1994). *Toxic Psychiatry*, St. Martin's Press, New York, pp. 95–6.
46. http://www.users.globalnet.co.uk/~drakb/schizophrenia.html
47. http://www.schizophrenia.com/news/causes2.html
48. http://www.schizophrenia.com/news/causes2.html
49. Sweeney, J. A., Haas, G. L., Keilp, J. G. and Long, M. (1991). Evaluation of the stability of neuropsychological functioning after acute episodes of schizophrenia: one-year follow-up study. *Psychiatry Research*, **38**, 63–76.
50. Breggin, P. R. (1994). *Toxic Psychiatry*, St. Martin's Press, New York, p. 116.
51. Leibrich, J. (1999). *A Gift of Stories: Discovering How to Deal with Mental Illness*, University of Otago Press, Dunedin.
52. Cohen, P. (2001). wysiwyg://8http://www.cedro-uva.org/lib/cohen.addiction.html
53. Abbott, M. W. and Walberg, R. A. (1999). Gambling and Problem Gambling Among Recently Sentenced Males in Four New Zealand Prisons, Wellington, Department of Internal Affairs.
54. American Psychiatric Association (2000). *Diagnostic and Statistical Manual of Mental Disorders* (Text Revision), Vol. IV. American Psychiatric Press, Washington, DC.
55. *International Journal of Mental Health Promotion*, passim.
56. Carnegie, D. (1994). *How to Win Friends and Influence People*, Hutchinson, London.
57. Gabor, D. (1985). *How to Start a Conversation and Make Friends*, Sheldon Press, Cambridge.
58. Friedman, M. (1999). *Reconsidering Logical Positivism*, Cambridge University Press.
59. Jahoda, M. (1958). *Current Concepts of Positive Mental Health*, Basic Books, New York.
60. Seedhouse, D. F. (1991). *Liberating Medicine*, John Wiley, Chichester.
61. Tenglend, P.-A. (1998). *Mental Health: A Philosophical Analysis*, Linköping Studies in Arts and Science, Linköping University, Sweden.

62. Downie, R. S., Fyfe, C. and Tannahill, A. (1990). *Health Promotion: Models and Values*, Oxford University Press, Oxford.
63. Seedhouse, D. F. (1997). *Health Promotion: Philosophy, Prejudice and Practice*, John Wiley, Chichester.
64. Redlich, F. and Freedman, D. (1966). *The Theory and Practice of Psychiatry*, Basic Books, London.
65. Cox, R. (1974). *American Handbook in Psychiatry*. [Sic] Incomplete reference, found in (Tenglend, ref. 61 above), p. 37.
66. Maslow, A. H. (1987). In R. Frager (ed.), *Motivation and Personality*, (3rd edn), Longman, London.
67. Jahoda, M. (1958). *Current Concepts of Positive Mental Health*, Basic Books, New York, p. 29.
68. Jahoda, M. (1958). *Current Concepts of Positive Mental Health*, Basic Books, New York, p. 46.
69. Lamb, T. and Bourriau, J. (eds) (1995). *Colour: Art and Science*, Cambridge University Press, Cambridge.
70. Graff, K. (1991). *Wave Motion in Elastic Solids*, Dover Publications, Mineola, NY.
71. Hawking, S. (2001). *The Universe in a Nutshell*, Bantam Press, London.
72. Hawking, S. (1995). *A Brief History of Time*, Bantam Press, London.
73. Koestler, A. (1964). *The Sleepwalkers*, Arkana, London.
74. Samuel, D. (2000). *Memory*, Orion Paperbacks, Crow's Nest, Australia.
75. Clark, A. (2000). *A Theory of Sentience*, Clarendon Press, Oxford.
76. Dawkins, R. (1989). *The Selfish Gene*, Oxford Paperbacks, Oxford.
77. Feyerabend, P. (1993). *Against Method* (3rd edn), Verso, London.
78. Goleman, D. (1996). *Emotional Intelligence*, Bloomsbury, London.
79. Hofstadter, D. R. (1982). *The Mind's I*, Penguin, Harmondsworth.
80. Elliot, A. (2001). *Concepts of the Self*, Polity Press, Oxford.
81. Seedhouse, D. F. (1998). Mental Health Promotion: Problems and Possibilities, *International Journal of Mental Health Promotion*, **1**:1, 5–14.
82. Damasio, A. (1994). *Descartes' Error*, Grosset/Putnam, New York, p. 10.
83. Damasio, A. (1994). *Descartes' Error*, Grosset/Putnam, New York, p. 134.
84. Damasio, A. (1994). *Descartes' Error*, Grosset/Putnam, New York, p. 200.
85. Damasio, A. (1994). *Descartes' Error*, Grosset/Putnam, New York, p. 173.
86. Glasson, J., Therivel, R. and Chadwick, A. (1998). *Introduction to Environmental Impact Assessment*, UCL Press, London.
87. Gleick, J. (1997). *Chaos*, Minerva, London.
88. Chakraborty, A. (1996). *Mind–body Dualism: A Philosophical Investigation*, D. K. Print World, India.
89. Rosenthal, D. (1987). *Materialism and the Mind-Body Problem*, Hackett Publishing Company, Indianapolis.
90. http://www.artsci.wustl.edu/~philos/MindDict/materialism.html
91. Stevens, R. (ed.) (1995). *Understanding the Self*, Sage, Thousand Oaks, CA.
92. Barnes, P. (1995). *Personal, Social and Emotional Development in Children*, Blackwell, Oxford.
93. Butler, J. (1999). *Gender Trouble*, Routledge, London.
94. http://www.mindbody.org/events/march_conference.html
95. Walton, J. A. (2000). Schizophrenia and Life in the World of Others, *Canadian Journal of Nursing Research*, **32**, 3, pp. 69–84.
96. http://healthhelper.com/complementary/book_mb/intro.htm
97. Pickering, T. G., James, G. D., Boddie, C. et al. (1988). How Common is White Coat Hypertension? *JAMA*, **259**, 225–228.
98. Seedhouse, D. F. (1998). *Ethics: the Heart of Health Care* (2nd edn), John Wiley, Chichester.
99. Simpson, G. G. (1953), p. 53: (quoted in http://healthhelper.com/complementary/book_mb/evidence.htm).
100. Koestler, A. (1979). *Janus: A Summing Up*, Pan Books, London.
101. Jarvie, I. C. (1970). Explaining Cargo Cults, in *Rationality*, ed. Bryan R. Wilson, Basil Blackwell, Oxford.
102. Jarvie, I. C. and Agassi, J. (1970). The Problem of the Rationality of Magic, in *Rationality*, ed. Bryan R. Wilson, Basil Blackwell, Oxford.
103. Kekes, I. (1976). *A Justification of Rationality*, Albany, State University of New York Press.

104. Seedhouse, D. F. (1984). *Rationality*, PhD Thesis, Manchester University (unpublished).
105. Camazine, S. (1992). *Self-organisation in Biological Systems*, Princeton University Press, Princeton, NJ.
106. Foulds, G. A. (1976). *Personal Illness*, Academic Press, London, p. 67.
107. Foulds G. A. (1976). *Personal Illness*, Academic Press, London, p. 93.
108. Smallwood, G. (1996). Aboriginality and Mental Health, in M. Clinton and S. Nelson (eds), *Mental Health and Nursing Practice*, Prentice-Hall, Sydney.
109. Feyerabend, P. (1991). *Three Dialogues on Knowledge*, Blackwell, Oxford.
110. Breggin, P. R. (1994). *Toxic Psychiatry*, St. Martin's Press, New York.
111. Laing, R. D. and Esterson, A. (1970). *Sanity, Madness and the Family*, Penguin Books, Harmondsworth.
112. Charlton, B. (2000). *Psychiatry and the Human Condition*, Lippincott, Williams and Wilkins, Philadelphia.
113. Trent, D. R. and Read, C. (eds) (1993). *Promotion of Mental Health*, Vol. 2, Avebury, Aldershot.
114. Trent, D. R. (ed.) (1992). *Promotion of Mental Health*, Vol. 1, Avebury, Aldershot.
115. Seedhouse, D. F. (2000). *Practical Nursing Philosophy: The Universal Ethical Code*, John Wiley, Chichester (Ch. 4: Dignity).
116. American Psychiatric Association (1994). *Diagnostic and Statistical Manual of Mental Disorders*, Vol. IV, pp. 354–5.
117. Hill, D. (1968). Depression: disease, reaction or posture? *American Journal of Psychiatry*, **125**, 445–57.
118. Bleuler, E. (1950). Dementia Praecox, International Universities Press, Madison, CT.
119. Foulds, G. A. (1976). *Personal Illness*, Academic Press, London, p. 106.
120. Foulds, G. A. (1976). *Personal Illness*, Academic Press, London, p. 11.
121. Foulds, G. A. (1976). *Personal Illness*, Academic Press, London, p. 106.
122. Hallowell, Edward M. and Ratey, John J. *Driven to Distraction* – referenced in Blumenfeld, S. (1999). *Homeschooling: A Parent's Guide to Teaching Children*, Replica Books, Bridgewater, NJ.
123. Blumenfeld, S. (1999). *Homeschooling: A Parent's Guide to Teaching Children*, Replica Books, Bridgewater, NJ.
124. http://www.mhc.govt.nz/mhc_PapersSp.htm
125. Gelder, M., Mayou, R. and Cowen, P. (2001). *The Shorter Oxford Textbook of Psychiatry* (4th edn), Oxford University Press, Oxford.
126. Steadman, H. J., McCarty, D. W. and Morrissey, J. P. (1989). *The Mentally Ill in Jail*, Guilford Press, New York.
127. Seedhouse, D. F. (2001). *Health: The Foundations for Achievement* (2nd edn), John Wiley, Chichester.
128. Brackx, Anny and Grimshaw, Catherine (eds) (1989). *Mental Health Care in Crisis*, Pluto Press, London.
129. Spence, R. and Johnston, P. (2001). *Oncology*, Oxford University Press, Oxford.
130. Souhami, R. et al. (2001). *Oxford Textbook of Oncology*, Oxford University Press, Oxford.
131. Casciato, D. A. (2000). *Manual of Clinical Oncology*, Lippincott, Williams and Wilkins, Philadelphia.
132. http://www.immunisation.org.uk/
133. http://www.new-atlantean.com/options.htm
134. Maclaren, P. and Seedhouse, D. (2001). Computer Mediated Communication with Integrated Graphical Tools Used For Health Care Decision Making, in G. Kennedy, M. Keppell, C. McNaught, T. Petrovvic (eds), *Short Paper Proceedings of the 18th Annual Conference of the Australasian Society for Computers in Learning in Tertiary Education* (ASCILITE) (pp. 109–112). The University of Melbourne, Australia. Paper available: http://www.ascilite.org.au/conferences/melbourne01/pdf/papers/maclarenp.pdf
135. http://www.hebs.scot.nhs.uk/services/mmr/pdf/MMRquestion6.pdf
136. World Health Organisation (1993). *Health for All Targets: The Health Policy for Europe*, European Health for All Series, No. 4, ISBN 92–890–13117.
137. Skrabanek, P. (1994). The Ethics of Prevention, in J. Le Fanu (ed.), *Preventionitis: The Exaggerated Claims of Health Promotion*, St. Edmundsbury Press, Suffolk, UK.

Index

Note: page numbers in *italics* refer to figures